ESASO Course Series

Vol. 10

Series Editors

F. Bandello Milan

B. Corcóstegui Barcelona

Imaging Techniques

Volume Editors

José Cunha-Vaz Coimbra
Adrian Koh Singapore

97 figures, 58 in color, and 3 tables, 2018

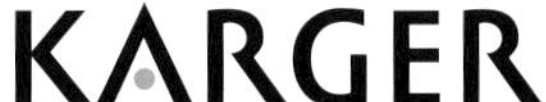

Basel · Freiburg · Paris · London · New York · Chennai · New Delhi ·
Bangkok · Beijing · Shanghai · Tokyo · Kuala Lumpur · Singapore · Sydney

José Cunha-Vaz
AIBILI – Association for Innovation and
Biomedical Research on Light and Image
Azinhaga de Santa Comba, Celas
3000-548 Coimbra (Portugal)
E-Mail cunhavaz@aibili.pt

Adrian Koh
Eye & Retina Surgeons
#13-03 Camden Medical Centre
1 Orchard Boulevard
Singapore 248649 (Singapore)
E-Mail ahckoh@yahoo.com

Library of Congress Cataloging-in-Publication Data

Names: Cunha-Vaz, Jose G., editor | Koh, Adrian, editor.
Title: Imaging techniques / volume editors, Jose Cunha-Vaz, Adrian Koh.
Other titles: ESASO course series ; v. 10. 1664-882X
Description: Basel ; New York : Karger, 2018. | Series: ESASO course series,
   ISSN 1664-882X ; vol. 10 | Includes bibliographical references and index.
Identifiers: LCCN 2018016821| ISBN 9783318063554 (hard cover : alk. paper) |
   ISBN 9783318063561 (electronic version)
Subjects: | MESH: Retinal Diseases--diagnostic imaging | Tomography, Optical
   Coherence | Fluorescein Angiography | Optical Imaging
Classification: LCC RE551 | NLM WW 270 | DDC 617.7/350754--dc23 LC record available at
https://lccn.loc.gov/2018016821

Contents

List of Contributors

Francesco Bandello, *p 52*
Department of Ophthalmology
University Vita Salute
IRCCS Ospedale San Raffaele
Via Olgettina, 60
20132 Milan (Italy)
E-Mail bandello.francesco@hsr.it

Adriano Carnevali, *p 52*
Department of Ophthalmology
University Vita Salute
IRCCS Ospedale San Raffaele
Via Olgettina 60, 20132 Milan (Italy)
E-Mail adrianocarnevali@live.it

Assoc. Prof. Gemmy C.M. Cheung, *p 1*
Singapore National Eye Center
11 Third Hospital Avenue
Singapore 168751 (Singapore)
E-Mail gemmy.cheung.c.m@singhealth.com.sg

José Cunha-Vaz, *p VIII, 88, 102*
AIBILI – Association for Innovation and
Biomedical Research on Light and Image
Azinhaga de Santa Comba, Celas
3000-548 Coimbra (Portugal)
E-Mail cunhavaz@aibili.pt

Federico Corvi, *p 102*
ASST Fatebenefratelli Sacco
Via G.B. Grassi, 74
20157 Milan (Italy)
E-Mail federico.corvi@yahoo.it

Monika Fleckenstein, *p 65*
University of Bonn
Department of Ophthalmology
Ernst-Abbe-Str. 2
53127 Bonn (Germany)
E-Mail monika.fleckenstein@ukbonn.de

K. Bailey Freund, *p 37*
Vitreous, Retina Macula
Consultants of New York
460 Park Ave, New York, NY 10022 (USA)
E-Mail kbfreund@gmail.com

Prof. Dr. Frank G. Holz, *p 65*
Department of Ophthalmology
University of Bonn
Ernst-Abbe-Strasse 2
53127 Bonn (Germany)
E-Mail Frank.Holz@ukbonn.de

Adrian Koh, *p VIII, 1*
Eye and Retina Surgeons
#13-03 Camden Medical Centre
1 Orchard Boulevard
Singapore 248649 (Singapore)
E-Mail ahckoh@yahoo.com

Inês Marques, *p 88*
AIBILI – Association for Innovation and
Biomedical Research on Light and Image
Azinhaga de Santa Comba, Celas
3000-548 Coimbra (Portugal)
E-Mail ipmarques@aibili.pt

Luis Mendes, *p 88*
AIBILI – Association for Innovation and
Biomedical Research on Light and Image
Azinhaga de Santa Comba, Celas
3000-548 Coimbra (Portugal)
E-Mail lgmendes@aibili.pt

Wei Kiong Ngo, *p 19*
National Healthcare Group Eye Institute
Tan Tock Seng Hospital
11 Jalan Tan Tock Seng
Singapore 308433 (Singapore)
E-Mail wkngo@hotmail.com

Maximilian Pfau, *p 65*
University of Bonn
Department of Ophthalmology
Ernst-Abbe-Str. 2
53127 Bonn (Germany)
E-Mail maximilian.pfau@ukbonn.de

Prof. Giuseppe Querques, *p 52*
Department of Ophthalmology
University Vita-Salute
IRCCS Ospedale San Raffaele
Via Olgettina 60, 20132 Milan (Italy)
E-Mail giuseppe.querques@hotmail.it

Lea Querques, *p 52*
Department of Ophthalmology
University Vita Salute
IRCCS Ospedale San Raffaele
Via Olgettina 60, 20132 Milan (Italy)
E-Mail lea_querques@hotmail.com

Riccardo Sacconi, *p 52*
Department of Ophthalmology
University Vita Salute
IRCCS Ospedale San Raffaele
Via Olgettina 60, 20132 Milan (Italy)
E-Mail ric.sacconi@gmail.com

Srinivas R. Sadda, *p 19*
Doheny Eye Institute
1355 San Pablo Street
Los Angeles, CA 90033 (USA)
E-Mail ssadda@doheny.org

Steffen Schmitz-Valckenberg, *p 65*
University of Bonn
Department of Ophthalmology
Ernst-Abbe-Str. 2
53127 Bonn (Germany)
E-Mail steffen.schmitz-valckenberg@ukbonn.de

Giovanni Staurenghi, *p 102*
ASST Fatebenefratelli Sacco
Via G.B. Grassi, 74
20157 Milan (Italy)
E-Mail giovanni.staurenghi@unimi.it

Anna C.S. Tan, *p 37*
Singapore National Eye Center
11 Third Hospital Avenue
Singapore 168751 (Singapore)
E-Mail annacstan@gmail.com

Colin S. Tan, *p 19*
National Healthcare Group Eye Institute
Tan Tock Seng Hospital
11 Jalan Tan Tock Seng
Singapore 308433 (Singapore)
E-Mail colintan_eye@yahoo.com.sg

Lawrence A. Yannuzzi, *p 37*
Vitreous, Retina Macula
Consultants of New York
460 Park Ave, New York, NY 10022 (USA)
E-Mail layannuzzi@gmail.com

Ilaria Zucchiatti, *p 52*
Department of Ophthalmology
University Vita Salute
IRCCS Ospedale San Raffaele
Via Olgettina 60, 20132 Milan (Italy)
E-Mail ilaria.zucchiatti@gmail.com

Preface

Ashton, who has contributed so extensively to our knowledge of retinal disease, remarked in 1974 that "we must continue to look for more fundamental scientific investigations and at the same time develop new ways of examining the retina in an effort to unravel the still unsolved questions". At that time most advances were based on histopathological studies using post-mortem material.

Since then, the advent of a variety of imaging modalities has completely changed the field and has brought retina examination and understanding of retinal disease from the laboratory in the daily clinical practice. It is possible now to follow retinal diseases in the consulting room almost at histopathological level. The decisions to treat are made now with much more confidence. The increase in knowledge in this area is tremendous and continuous. I can say that imaging is at the center of eye disease diagnosis and management.

Fundus photography and angiography has now improved much and the contribution of new techniques particularly with wide-field examinations are reviewed in the first chapter.

The second chapter addressed Optical Coherence Tomography. The relevance of this method is unique and is constantly offering new perspectives, allowing both qualitative and quantitative analysis of the choroidal and retinal tissues.

The third chapter focuses on Choroidal Imaging using optical coherence tomography. This is an emerging field that has brought new perspectives to the forgotten role of the choroid on choroid retinal disease.

The fourth chapter reviews Optical Coherence Angiography, a relatively new non-invasive method of studying the choroidal and retinal circulations.

The fifth chapter analyses the subject of autofluorescence imaging. Fundus autofluorescence allows for mapping of physiological and pathological fluorophores of the ocular fundus. It is a challenging but also extremely promising area.

Finally, the last chapters are dedicated to multimodal imaging. The availability of the previously described imaging modalities offers tremendous potential particularly when used in combination. Information from different imaging modalities add upon each other and offer entirely new perspectives allowing better information in each individual patient.

This book is seen not only as an update on the different imaging modalities, but also as an information source for those that are using imaging in their daily practice and want to understand fully what they see for the benefit of their patients.

José Cunha-Vaz, Coimbra
Adrian Koh, Singapore

Cunha-Vaz J, Koh A (eds): Imaging Techniques.
ESASO Course Series. Basel, Karger, 2018, vol 10, pp 1–18 (DOI: 10.1159/000487409)

Fundus Photography and Angiography

Gemmy C.M. Cheung[a, b] · Adrian Koh[a, c]

[a]Singapore Eye Research Institute, Singapore National Eye Centre, Singapore, [b]Duke NUS Graduate Medical School, Singapore, and [c]Eye and Retina Associates, Singapore, Singapore

Abstract

Fundus photography and angiography have become an integral part of the management of many retinal conditions, including age-related macular degeneration, diabetic retinopathy, retinal vascular diseases, as well as chorioretinal inflammatory conditions. In this chapter, we will review the clinical utility of these imaging modalities with illustrated examples in a range of common retinal conditions. Recent advances, including widefield photography and angiography, videoangiography and confocal scanning laser ophthalmoscopy-based angiography will be introduced, with illustrative examples of their clinical utility. Color fundus photography (CFP) is a useful tool to document changes in the retina and optic nerve. In the clinic setting, CFP is particularly useful to document baseline findings and facilitate longitudinal comparison. Angiography is a more detailed evaluation which assesses both the intravascular and extravascular compartments of the retina and choroid, usually after an intravenous injection of a fluorescent dye. This guides in the diagnosis, localization, and treatment of various diseases of the choroid and retina. Fluorescein angiography and indocyanine green angiography are the two most commonly used dyes for fundus angiography.

Color Fundus Photography

Color fundus photography (CFP) has been widely used in clinical practice as well as in research and population screening. CFP is an effective imaging modality to document changes in the posterior pole (Fig. 1). Montage of several images

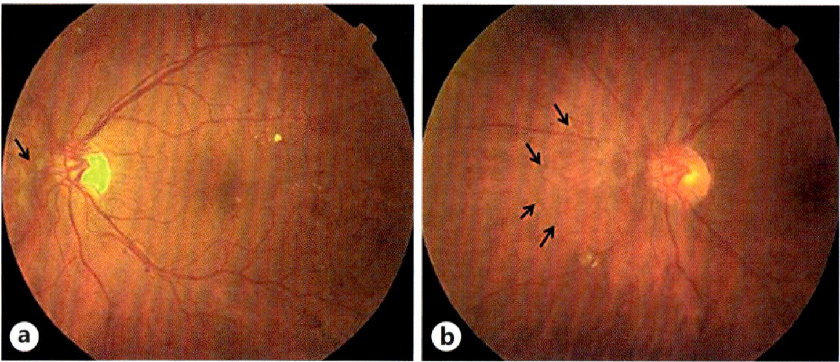

Fig. 1. Color fundus photography of an eye with proliferative diabetic retinopathy. Image centered on fovea (**a**) shows neovascularization at the disc (NVD; arrows) as well as areas of dot and blot hemorrhages and hard exudates. NVD can be seen more clearly on the image centered on the disc (**b**).

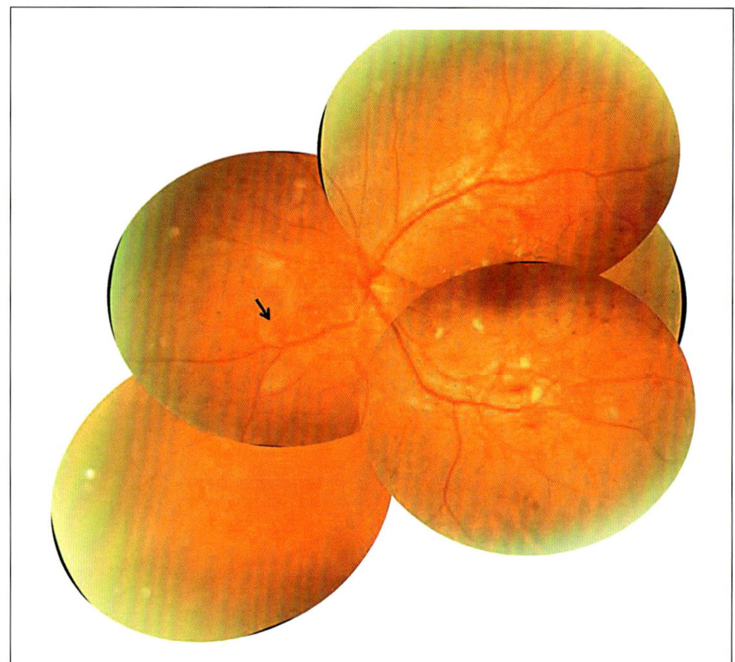

Fig. 2. Montage of color photographs to document posterior pole as well as peripheral retina. In this montage of an eye with severe nonproliferative diabetic retinopathy, widespread dot, blot, and flame hemorrhages, as well as cotton wool spots can be seen. Intraretinal microvascular abnormality can be seen in the nasal retina (arrow).

capturing the periphery of the retina can further provide the basis for assessment of the periphery of the retina (Fig. 2). Early Treatment Diabetic Retinopathy Study (ETDRS) 7-standard field 35-mm 30° stereoscopic CFP has been widely accepted as the gold standard for evaluation of severity of diabetic retinopathy (DR). Based on CFP, the severity of DR can be determined by grading the degree of the following lesions according to the modified Airlie House classification [1]: hemorrhages, microaneurysms (MAs), intraretinal microvascular abnormalities, venous beading, cotton wool spots, hard exudates, retinal thickening, neovascularization, preretinal hemorrhage, vitreous hemorrhage, and traction retinal detachment. A combination of ETDRS field 1 (centered on disc) and field 2 (centered on fovea) has been adopted for population screening of DR [2]. Subsequent studies have reported good to excellent agreement between film and digital images in determining DR severity.

High-quality stereoscopic CFP has also been widely used to assess the severity of age-related macular degeneration (AMD), typically using

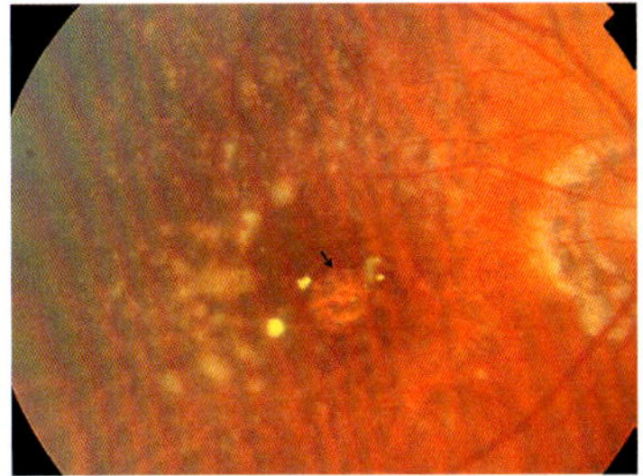

Fig. 3. Color fundus photography of any eye with age-related macular degeneration. Extensive drusen of variable sizes, some confluent, can be seen throughout the macula. An area of geographic atrophy can also be seen (arrow), characterized by the well-circumscribed round shape within which the underlying choroidal vessels can clearly be seen.

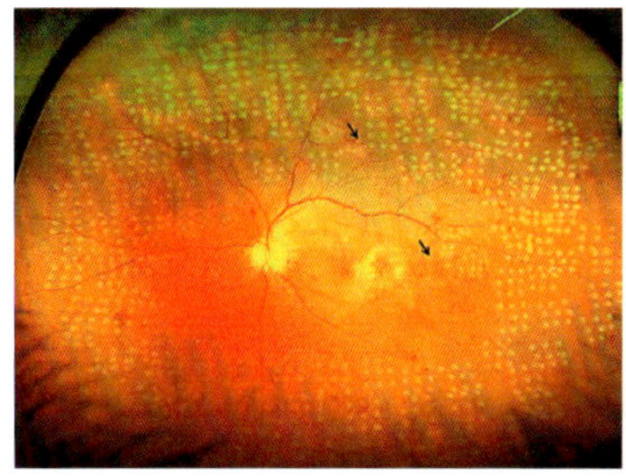

Fig. 4. Ultrawide-field photograph of an eye with proliferative diabetic retinopathy and diabetic macular edema. Multiple areas of new vessels elsewhere can be seen (arrows). There are hard exudates and microaneurysms at the macula. Panretinal photocoagulation laser burns can be seen.

modifications of the Wisconsin AMD grading system [3]. This method has been employed in many population-based studies around the world, including the Beaver Dam and Blue Mountains Eye Studies [4]. Features assessed include drusen characteristics as well as pigmentary changes for early AMD, whereas signs of pigment epithelial detachment (PED), choroidal neovascularization (CNV), and geographic atrophy are the key features assessed for late AMD (Fig. 3). Detailed grading of early AMD features of drusen characteristics based on CFP, include drusen size (usually graded categorically as small <63 μm; ≥63 and <125 μm; ≥125 and <250 μm; ≥250 μm), drusen border (distinct vs. indistinct), characteristics (soft, calcified, or reticular), plus total drusen area. In longitudinal studies, drusen area and drusen size were identified as important indicators of AMD progression [5, 6].

Widefield Photography

The ETDRS photography protocol is estimated to cover only 30% of the entire retinal surface. Lesions in the peripheral retina may not be fully evaluated even with ETDRS standard 7-field photographs. Ultrawide-field (UWF) retinal im-

aging systems using scanning laser ophthalmoscope technology combined with a large ellipsoidal mirror allows imaging of up to 90° of the retina in a single image without the need for pupil dilation. This is estimated to cover 82% of the entire retina surface (Fig. 4). Previous comparative studies have demonstrated a high degree of agreement between UWF photography and ETDRS film photographs. In addition, UWF enables more peripheral lesions to be detected, leading to an estimated reclassification of DR in 10% of eyes [7, 8]. UWF photography is also valuable in the follow-up of peripheral retinal pathologies, such as viral retinitis (Fig. 5), peripheral vascular diseases (Fig. 6), and retinal degeneration and tears.

Principles behind Fluorescein and Indocyanine Green Angiography

Conventional angiography exploits the different properties of dyes during various phases of the angiogram to evaluate the integrity of retinal and choroidal vasculature, and of the condition of the retinal pigment epithelium (RPE). After an intravenous injection of a bolus of dye, fluorescence can be detected within the choroid, followed by

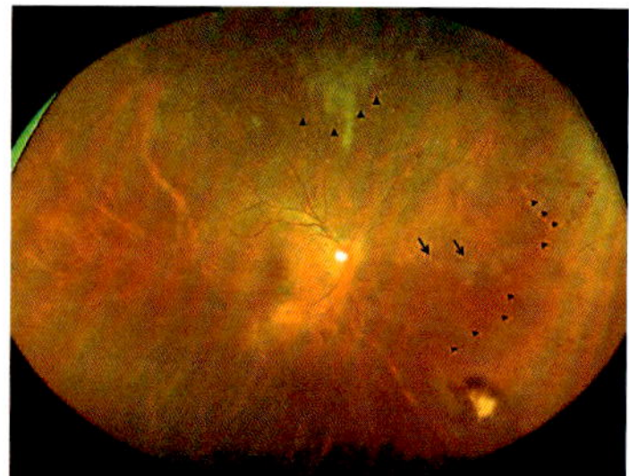

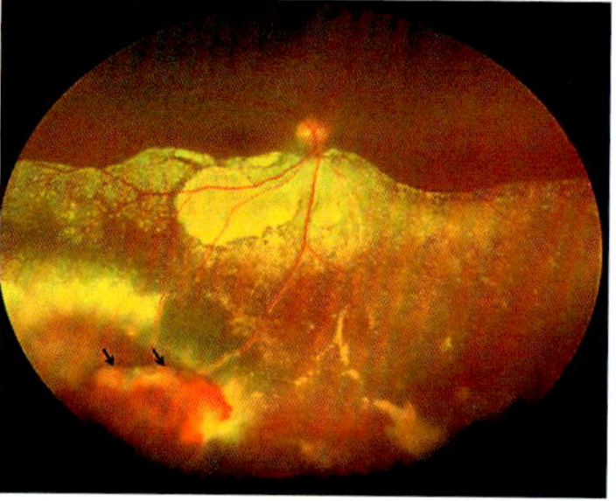

Fig. 5. Ultrawide-field photograph of an eye with acute retinal necrosis due to herpes zoster. The overall image is cloudy due to moderate vitritis. However, peripheral retinal necrosis can be seen as areas of retinal whitening (arrowheads). Attenuation and sclerosis of the peripheral retinal arterioles can also be seen, signifying arteritis (arrows).

Fig. 6. Ultrawide-field photograph of an eye with extensive exudation resulting from retinal angioma in the inferior retina (arrows).

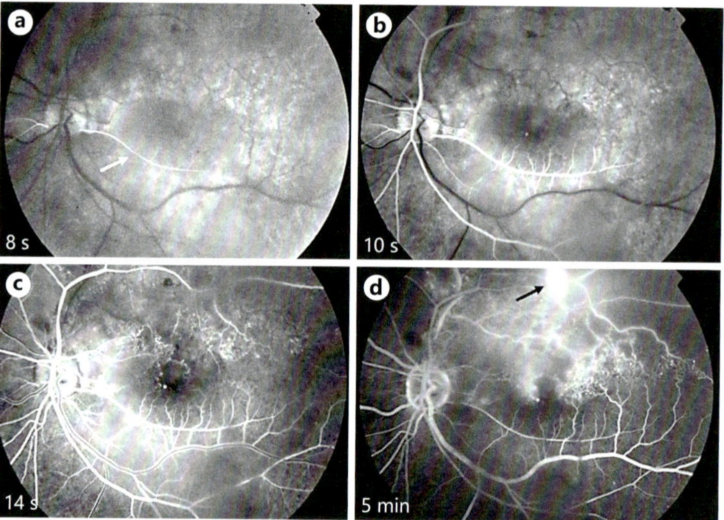

Fig. 7. Fluorescein angiography of an eye with superotemporal retinal vein occlusion. Choroidal flush and presence of a cilioretinal artery (white arrow) can be seen in the 8-s frame (**a**). This is followed by filling of the central retinal artery 2 s later (**b**). Laminar flow within the retina veins except in the superotemporal branch can be seen in the 14-s frame (arteriovenous phase; **c**), confirming the diagnosis. In the late frame taken at 5 min (**d**), nonperfusion of the superotemporal retina and disruption of the foveal avascular zone can be seen. Leakage from an area of neovascularization can be seen (black arrow).

the retina arterial and venous circuit within 5–30 s (transit-phase images). After complete filling of the retinal vein, the dye begins to be recirculated (midphase images). After 5 min (and up to 20–30 min) of recirculation, late-phase images are acquired (Fig. 7). The key differences between fluorescein and indocyanine green are summarized in Table 1 (Fig. 8).

Fluorescence from the dye should appear promptly within the choroidal and retinal vasculature in healthy eyes and not leak. However, hyperfluorescence may appear due to a window defect as a result of RPE atrophy, staining (such as in drusen or optic disc), pooling within a serous retinal detachment, or leakage through diseased vasculature. Conversely, hypofluorescence may result from masking by overlying tissue or perfusion defects. Viewing of stereo-pairs of images acquired at slightly different angles allows appreciation of depth of various lesions and is particularly important in diagnosing certain conditions, such as retinal angiomatous proliferation (RAP)

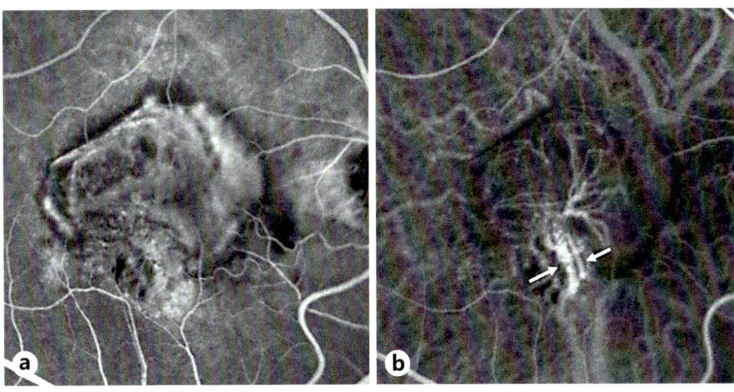

Fig. 8. Type 2 choroidal neovascularization (CNV) imaged on fluorescein (FA) and indocyanine green (ICGA) angiography. The CNV appears as hyperfluorescent network with leakage in the FA (**a**) but not in the ICGA (**b**). Feeder and draining vessels (arrows) are visible on the ICGA but not on the FA.

Table 1. Key differences between fluorescein and indocyanine green

	Fluorescein	Indocyanine green
Molecule	Small (molecular weight, 376 Da) 80% bound	Large (molecular weight, 775 Da) 98% plasma protein bound
Emission range	530 nm (green) Masked by RPE, thick blood and fibrotic tissue	790–805 nm (near infrared) Penetrates through RPE
Leakage	Leaks readily through abnormal vasculature	Minimal leak
Main utility	Assessing retinal vasculature and lesions above the RPE, e.g. – Diabetic retinopathy – Retinal vascular diseases – Choroidal neovascularization	Assessing choroidal vasculature, e.g. – Polypoidal choroidal vasculopathy – Choroidal inflammation – Choroidal tumors

and polypoidal CNV. In addition to still images, videoangiography allows for assessment of the dynamic features, including the filling pattern, speed, and pulsations within the vessels.

Neovascular Age-Related Macular Degeneration

Neovascular AMD typically presents with hemorrhage and swelling of the macula. In chronic lesions, hard exudate and fibrosis may also develop. These lesion components can be documented with CFP, fluorescein angiography (FA), and indocyanine green angiography (ICGA). FA is widely considered as the gold standard for diagnosis of neovascular AMD. Two patterns of leakage are generally described: classic and occult.

Classic pattern (Fig. 9) appears as a well-defined hyperfluorescent lesion in the early phase of the angiogram, often with a "lacy" pattern, which leaks (increases in intensity and size) in the late phase. This appearance is explained by the presence of the CNV above the RPE (type 2 CNV).

Occult pattern (Fig. 10) appears either as fibrovascular PED, which appears as an area of elevated, stippled hyperfluorescence when viewed stereoscopically, or as late leakage of unknown origin. This appearance results from CNV growing beneath the RPE (type 1 CNV). Type 1 CNVs are often associated with a serous PED which appears as a well-circumscribed dome-shaped ele-

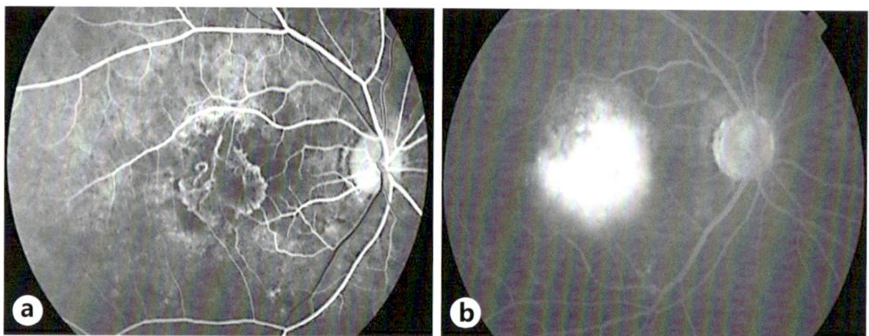

Fig. 9. Type 2 choroidal neovascularization on fluorescein angiography. In the early arteriovenous phase (**a**), a hyperfluorescent network with lacy pattern can be seen clearly. In the late phase (**b**), profuse leakage can be seen, as evident from the increase in intensity and size of the area of hyperfluorescence, extending beyond the margin of the network seen in the early phase.

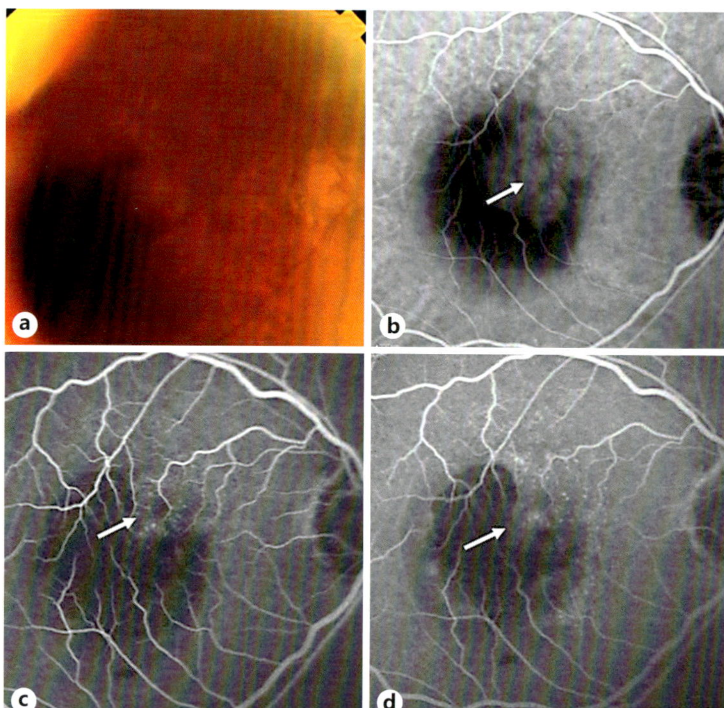

Fig. 10. Type 1 choroidal neovascularization. On color photograph (**a**), a dome-shaped elevation at the level of RPE can be seen. This area correspond to a pigment epithelial detachment which appears dark on ICGA (**b**) and FA (**c, d**). At the superior corner, a notch in the PED can be seen as stippled hyperfluorescence on FA with mild leakage, which suggests an area of fibrovascular PED. The corresponding area appears as a plaque on ICGA.

vation of the RPE in which dye can be seen to pool.

Type 3 CNV, also known as RAP originates from intraretinal neovascularization which progresses and extends beneath the neurosensory retina forming subretinal neovascularization and vascularized PED (Fig. 11). On FA, a focal area of early leakage with right-angled "diving vessel" may be seen. PEDs are commonly associated with stage 2 and 3 RAP. Dynamic angiography is valuable in determining the origin and direction of filling of the lesion [9].

CNV lesions can also be composed of a combination of the above lesions. "Predominantly classic" lesions are composed of >50% of classic CNV, whereas "Minimally classic" lesions are composed of <50% classic CNV. Other lesion components, such as thick blood or blocked fibrosis may appear as areas of hypofluorescence and staining respectively, and may obscure the

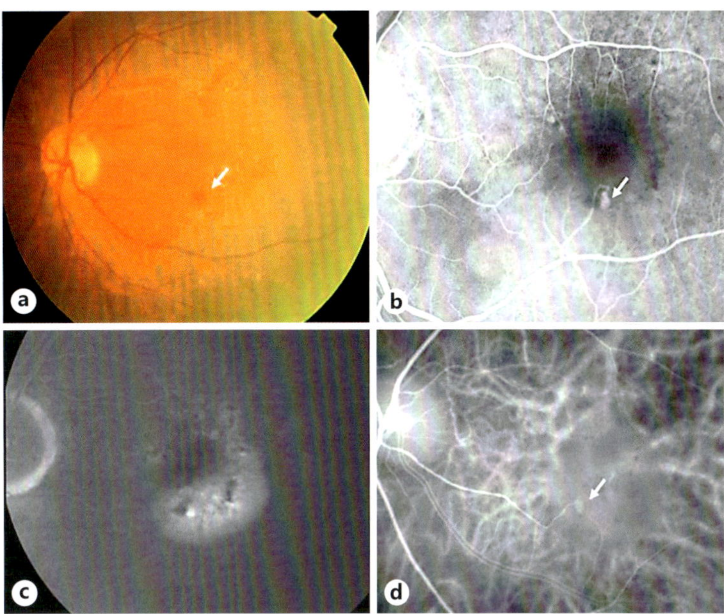

Fig. 11. Type 3 neovascularization (retinal angiomatous proliferation, RAP). On color photograph (**a**), a superficial hemorrhage can be seen on a background of reticular drusen. On the fluorescein angiogram (FA), the RAP lesion can be seen as an aneurysmal lesion (arrow) in the arteriovenous phase (**b**) which originates from anastomosis between two retinal vessels, with a characteristic "diving vessel" configuration. In the late-phase FA (**c**), a pigment epithelial detachment appears as a dome-shaped elevated area surrounding the RAP lesion. The RAP lesion appears as a hot spot on indocyanine angiography (**d**).

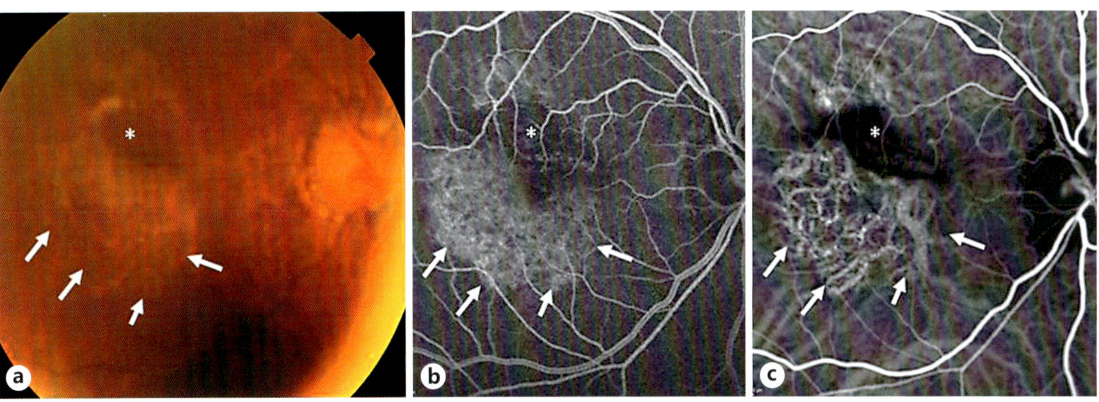

Fig. 12. Retinal pigment epithelial (RPE) tear. An RPE tear has developed in the eye with type 1 choroidal neovascularization in Figure 10. A round well-defined area of bearing of underlying choroidal vessels can be seen on color photograph (**a**) and appears as a window defect on the fluorescein angiogram (**b**) and indocyanine green angiogram (**c**). The stump of the torn RPE appears as a dark patch (*) at the superior border of the previously noted pigment epithelial detachment.

view of the underlying area which may harbor CNV. Tense PEDs may be complicated by RPE tear (Fig. 12). This may appear as submacular hemorrhage, often associated with a sudden drop in vision. RPE tears have a characteristic appearance on FA, which is helpful to make the diagnosis. The area devoid of RPE appears as a sharply demarcated area of hyperfluorescence which does not leak, due to unmasking of underlying choroidal vasculature. The stump of RPE typically appears dark, with variable leakage depending on whether the underlying CNV is

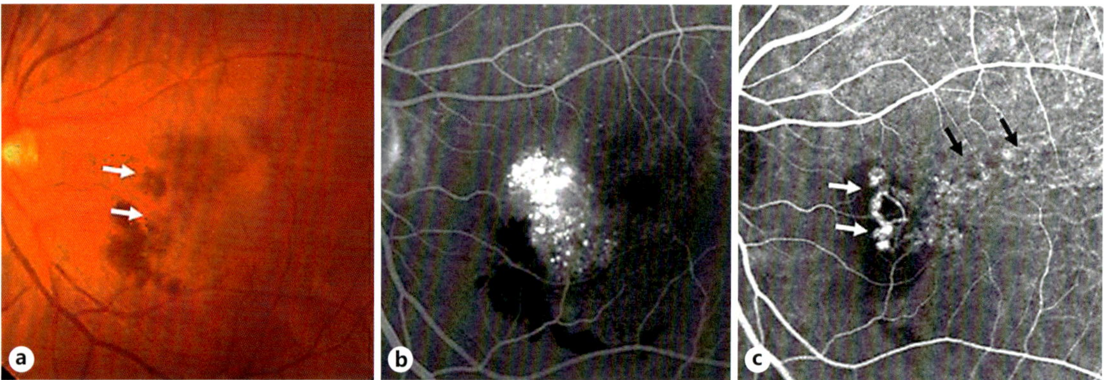

Fig. 13. Polypoidal choroidal vasculopathy. Orange subretinal nodules can be seen on color fundus photography (**a**) (white arrows). On fluorescein angiogram, the appearance of occult leakage pattern is indistinguishable from type 1 choroidal neovascularization (**b**). On indocyanine green angiography (**c**), however, a clear string of polyps (white arrows) can be identified, as well as a branching vascular network (black arrows).

still active. On ICGA, CNV lesions typically appear as a hot spot or plaque in the late phase (Fig. 10).

Polypoidal Choroidal Vasculopathy

Polypoidal choroidal vasculopathy (PCV) is widely considered a variant of type 1 CNV. PCV often presents as serosanguineous maculopathy and large submacular hemorrhage. The PCV lesion complex is often comprised of two parts: polyps and branching vascular network (BVN). Both components typically reside beneath the RPE [10, 11]. On FA, therefore, an occult leakage pattern is typically observed, and is often indistinguishable from type 1 CNV. On ICGA, however, polyps can be seen as focal hyperfluorescent lesions which are often nodular in appearance and appear within the first 6 min after dye injection (Fig. 13). Other associated features include the presence of BVN, hypofluorescent halo around the polyp, pulsatility on dynamic ICGA, or the association of orange subretinal nodule on color photograph or massive submacular hemorrhage. The confocal scanning laser ophthalmoscope (cSLO)-based ICGA platform can acquire

higher contrast images compared to flash-camera-based ICGA and has been shown to be superior at detecting BVN [12, 13]. A further advantage of the cSLO-based ICGA system is the ability to acquire videoangiography. This allows further assessment of the dynamic properties of the lesion, including speed and direction of filling. Features that are best evaluated using videoangiography include pulsatility, feeder vessels, and anastomotic vessels as in RAP.

DR and Diabetic Macular Edema

FA is a valuable imaging tool in the assessment of DR and diabetic macular edema (DME). In particular, FA can highlight MAs, areas of nonperfusion, and neovascularization, as well as assess the integrity of the foveal avascular zone and macular edema. New vessels can be differentiated from intraretinal microvascular abnormalities as the latter do not leak (Fig. 14). Widefield angiography is now available on several commercially available devices (Fig. 15). The detection of DME using CFP has limited specificity as this modality relies on an indirect assessment based on the detection of loss of retinal transparency, hard exudates, and

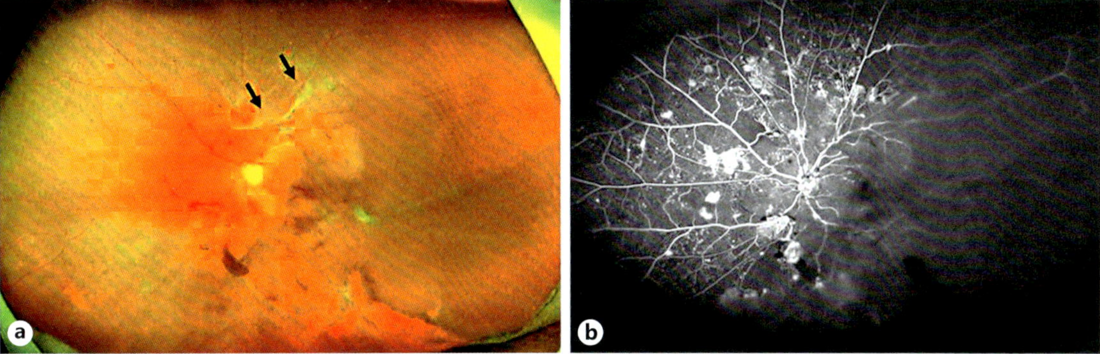

Fig. 14. Proliferative diabetic retinopathy. Ultrawide-field photography (**a**) and fluorescein angiography (**b**) showing preretinal hemorrhage, multiple areas of nonperfusion and neovascularization. On color photograph, an area of fibrosis and localized traction (arrows) can be seen in the superior retina. The view of the temporal retina is obscured by vitreous hemorrhage.

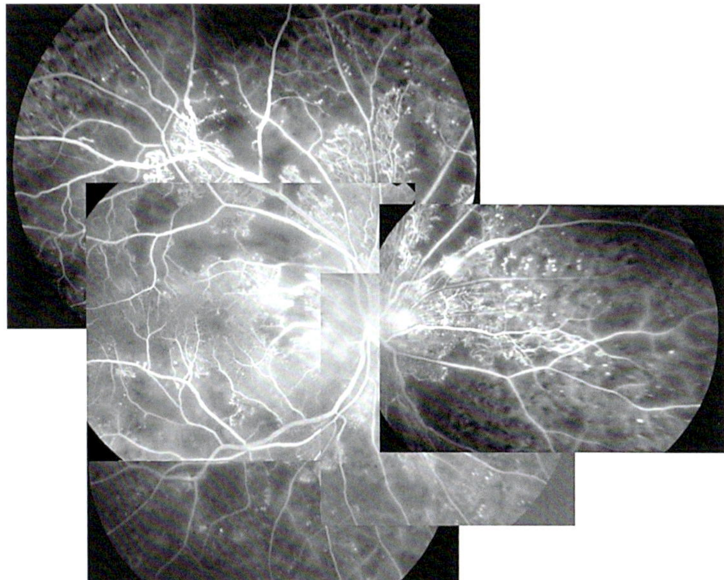

Fig. 15. Proliferative diabetic retinopathy with significant retinal nonperfusion. Montage of multiple 30° fluorescein angiography images can also provide information on the posterior pole as well as peripheral retina. Extensive areas of capillary nonperfusion, and areas of neovascularization can be seen in this eye.

MAs near the fovea, albeit without appreciation of macular thickening. Incorporation of optical coherence tomography (OCT) has greatly improved the sensitivity and specificity of DME detection. On FA, however, DME can be readily identified in the presence of late leakage. In addition, identifying the origin of leakage (focal from MAs or diffuse), is essential to guide targeted focal laser treatment [14] (Fig. 16).

Other Retinal Vascular Diseases

In eyes with retinal vein occlusion, FA can be used to confirm the site of occlusion, detect macular edema, and determine if there is macular or peripheral ischemia (Fig. 7, 17, 18). New vessels can be differentiated from collaterals as the latter do not leak. Widefield FA may identify areas of peripheral nonperfusion not readily visible on stan-

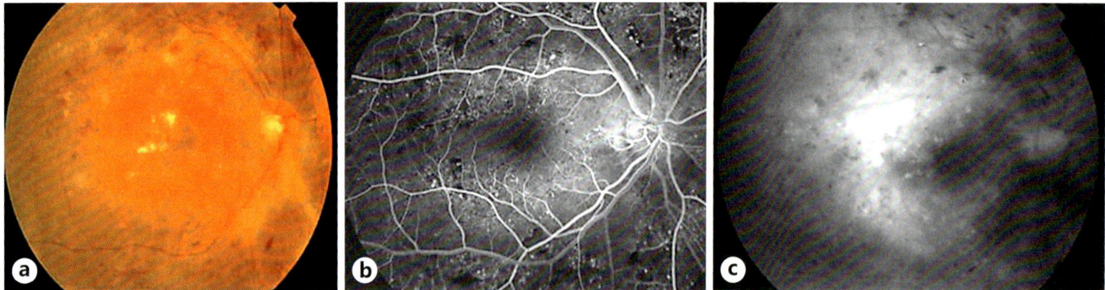

Fig. 16. Diabetic macular edema (DME). Microaneurysms and hard exudates can be seen within the macula on color photograph (**a**). The early-phase fluorescein angiogram (**b**) showed multiple microaneurysms and masking from blot hemorrhages. The foveal avascular zone appears relatively intact despite DME. Diffuse leakage is confirmed in the late-phase angiogram (**c**).

Fig. 17. Nonischemic central retinal vein occlusion. Widespread flame and blot hemorrhages as well as venous congestion can be seen on the color photograph (**a**). On the early-phase fluorescein angiogram (**b**), arteriole filling can be seen at 9 s. However arteriolar-venous filling was prolonged. Lamellar flow can still be seen within the retinal veins at 21 s (**c**). Foveal avascular zone was preserved. In the 6-min frame (**d**), staining of the optic disc and the superotemporal vein can be seen, but there was no significant macular edema.

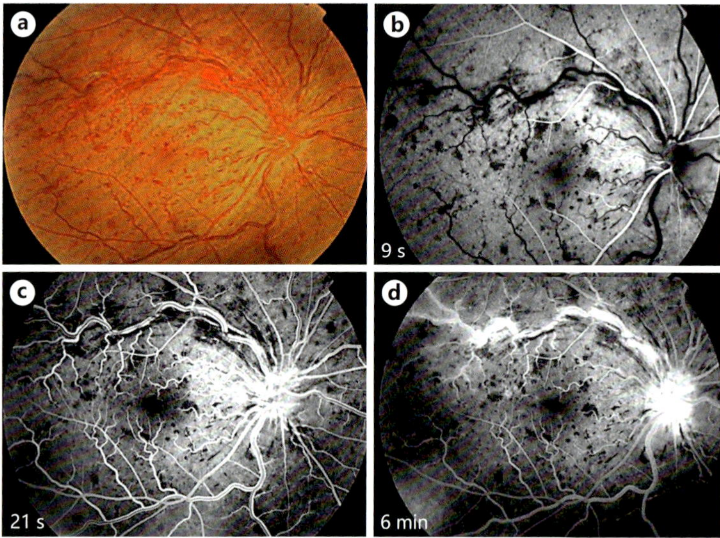

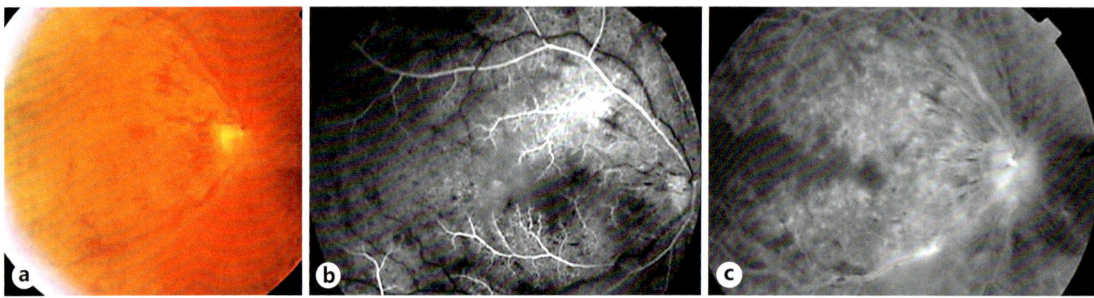

Fig. 18. Central retinal vein occlusion with macular ischemia. Scattered flame and blot hemorrhages can be seen on the color photograph (**a**). On the early-phase fluorescein angiogram (**b**), the foveal avascular zone appears enlarged and irregular. On the late-phase angiogram (**c**), a large area of nonperfusion is evident extending from the fovea towards the temporal retina. Staining of the optic disc and retinal veins can also be seen.

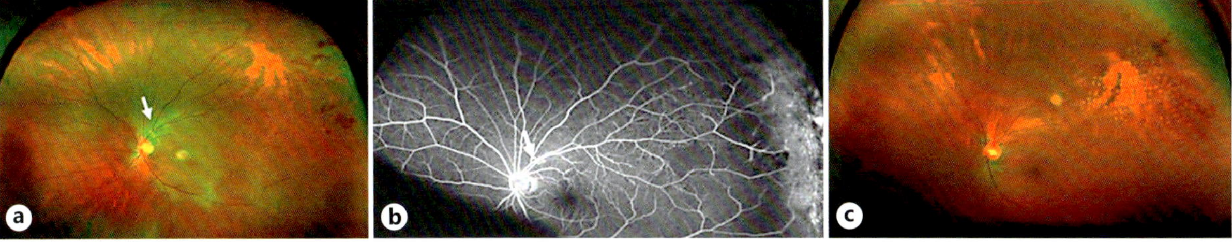

Fig. 19. Peripheral retinal nonperfusion secondary to superotemporal branch retinal vein occlusion. The superotemporal branch retinal vein is occluded beyond the arteriovenous crossing (arrow). No significant abnormality can be seen in the posterior pole. However, blot hemorrhages can be seen in the far periphery (**a**). Peripheral retinal nonperfusion can be seen in the corresponding location on the ultrawide-field fluorescein angiogram (**b**). Photocoagulation was performed targeting the areas of nonperfusion (**c**).

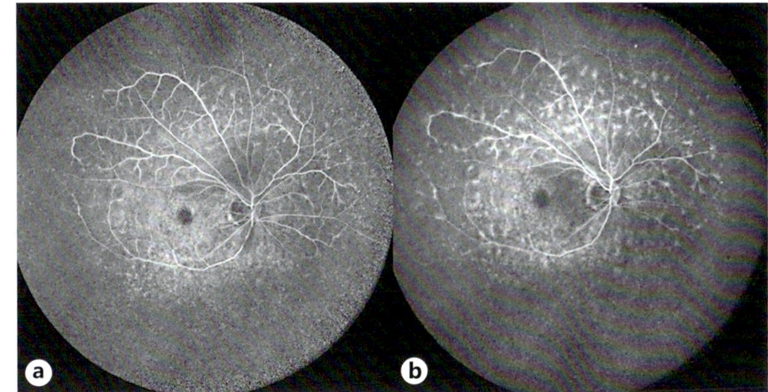

Fig. 20. Occlusive retinal vasculitis secondary to systemic lupus erythematosus. Early-phase fluorescein angiogram (**a**) showing pruning of peripheral vessels and extensive area of nonperfusion in the peripheral retina. Late-phase image (**b**) shows diffuse leakage indicating active vasculitis.

dard FA, and help guide laser treatment to ischemic areas (Fig. 19).

Other retinal vascular diseases in which FA is useful include retinal vasculitis (Fig. 20), Coat's disease (Fig. 21), Eales' disease (Fig. 22), radiation retinopathy (Fig. 23), and retinal angioma. In order to acquire the most relevant information, very early transit-phase images are particularly important for investigating choroidal circulation, retinal arteriolar occlusion, and cilioretinal artery perfusion. For evaluation of peripheral areas, peripheral images should be taken in order to produce a montage. Alternatively, UWF angiography can provide information on up to 200° of view in a single image.

Central Serous Chorioretinopathy

Central serous chorioretinopathy (CSC) is characterized by detachment of the neurosensory retina, often with PED. In acute CSC, FA may identify the source of focal leakage in the form of "smokestack" or "inkblot" appearance (Fig. 24). Pooling from associated PEDs may also be seen. Focal laser to these leakage points, if located extrafoveally, may hasten the resolution of the neurosensory detachment. Where leakage areas are extensive, photodynamic therapy may be preferred. In chronic or recurrent CSC, FA, together with fundus autofluorescence, can also demonstrate the extent of RPE damage which appears as a window defect. These areas

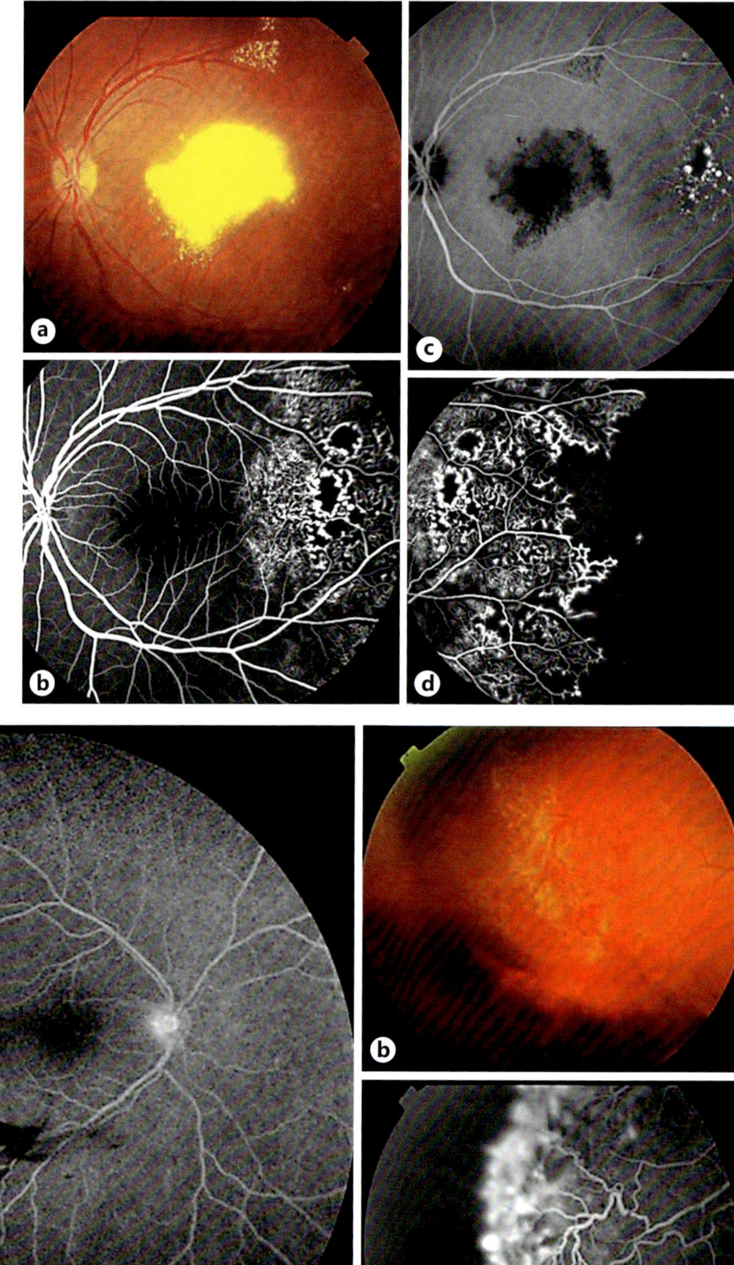

Fig. 21. Coat's disease. On color photograph (**a**), a large plaque made up of hard exudates can be seen in the macula. On the fluorescein angiogram (**b**, **d**), telangiectatic vessels and peripheral nonperfusion can be seen in the temporal retina. The aneurysmal dilatations are clearly seen on the indocyanine green angiogram (**c**).

Fig. 22. Eales' disease. On the widefield fluorescein angiogram (**a**), preretinal hemorrhage can be seen along the inferotemporal arcade. An area of neovascularization with intense leakage can be seen in the periphery. Details of neovascularization can be seen on images with higher magnification (**b**, **c**).

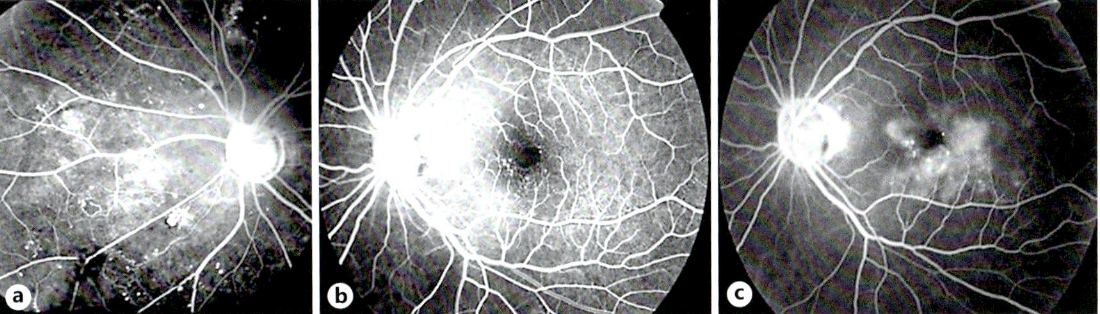

Fig. 23. Radiation retinopathy. Many features of radiation retinopathy are similar to changes in diabetic retinopathy. On this fluorescein angiogram of a patient who had previously undergone radiation for nasopharyngeal carcinoma, microaneurysms can be seen in the nasal retina (**a**) and enlargement of the foveal avascular zone in the posterior pole (**b**). Leakage indicating macular edema can be seen on the late-phase image (**c**).

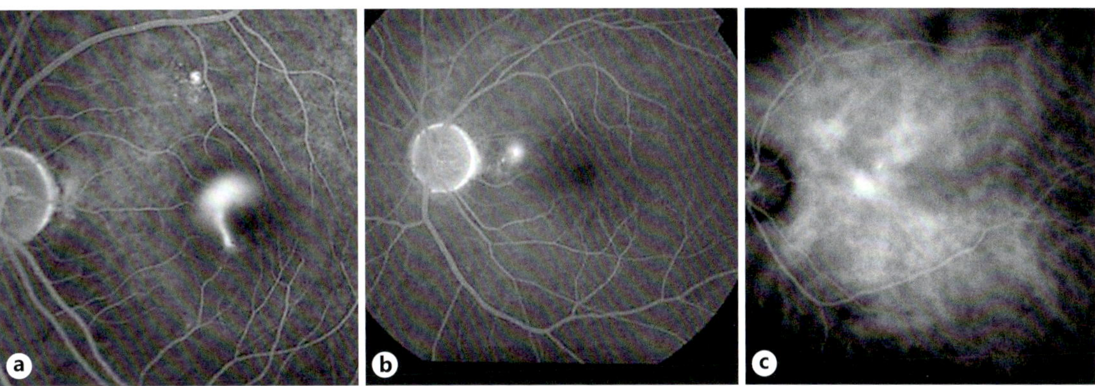

Fig. 24. Acute central serous chorioretinopathy (CSC). Typical appearance of fluorescein angiogram in acute CSC is focal leak at the level of the retinal pigment epithelium in the form of smokestack (**a**) or inkblot (**b**) pattern. Choroidal hyperpermeability is often present and is best seen on indocyanine angiogram (**c**).

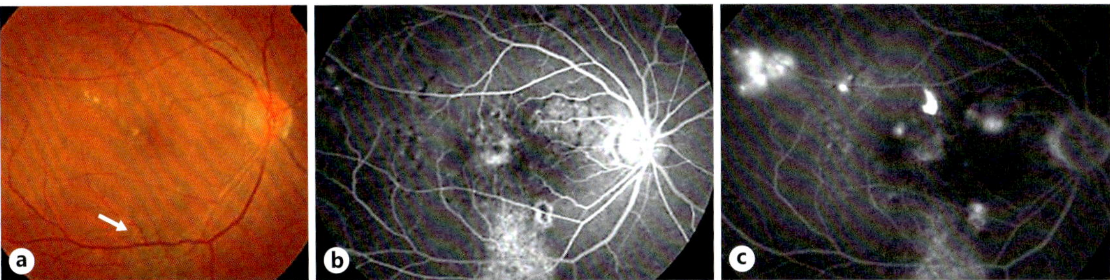

Fig. 25. Chronic central serous chorioretinopathy. Extensive mottling of the retinal pigment epithelium in the pattern of a "downward track" can be seen on the color photograph (arrow; **a**). This area appears as irregular window defects on the fluorescein angiogram (**b**). In addition, some areas of pinpoint leakage are still visible (**c**).

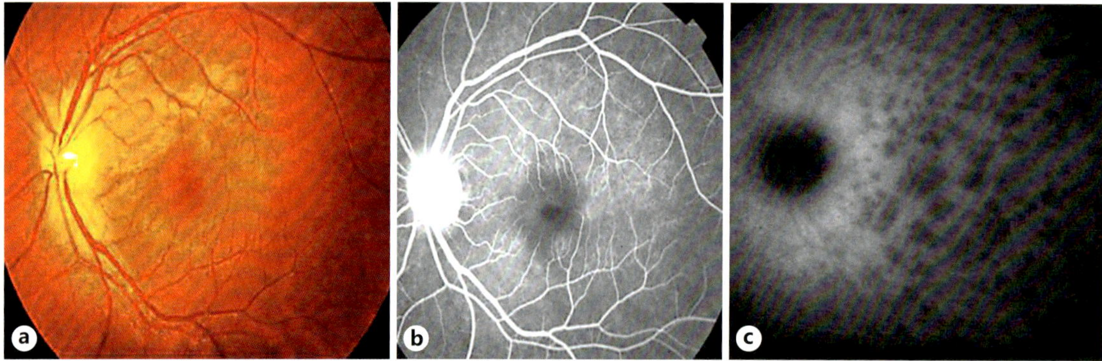

Fig. 26. Multiple evancescent white dot syndrome. This 28-year-old lady had a history of recent-onset central scotoma with photopsia. The appearance of the posterior pole was unremarkable (**a**). Disc hyperfluorescence is seen on late-phase fluorescein angiogram (**b**). Multiple hypofluorescent spots are seen on the indocyanine green angiogram (**c**).

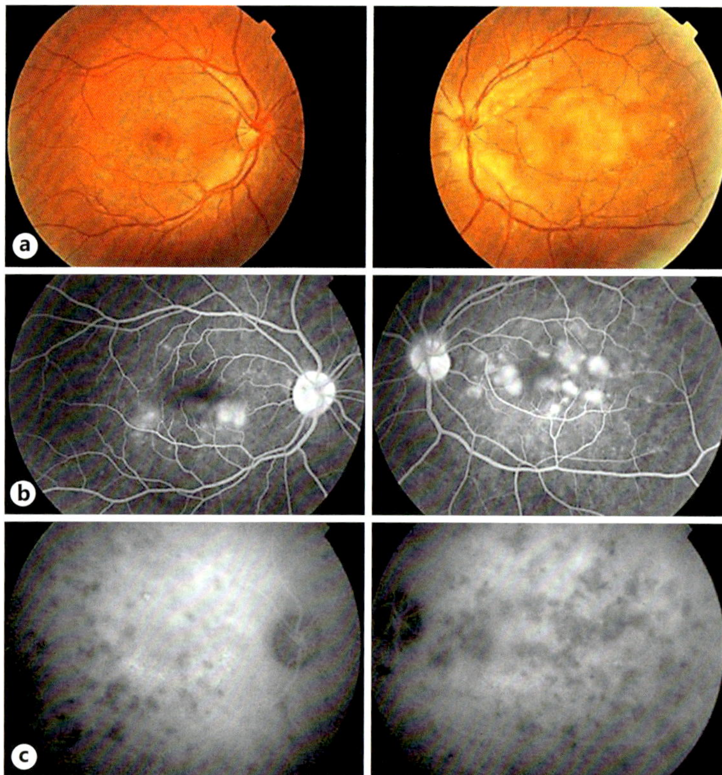

Fig. 27. Vogt-Koyanagi-Harada disease. Typical features include multiple neurosensory detachments affecting both eyes (**a**). On fluorescein angiogram, pinpoint hyperfluorescent dots at the level of the retinal pigment epithelium are visible in the early phase which continue to leak and eventually pool into areas of serous detachment (**b**). On indocyanine green angiogram (**c**), multiple hypofluorescent dark dots can be seen which are believed to represent choroidal nonperfusion. In addition, fuzziness of the large choroidal vessels can be seen.

may appear as a "downward gravitational track" in chronic cases (Fig. 25). This information is important in prognosticating visual outcome. Choroidal vascular hyperpermeability is often noted in CSC and is best visualized with ICGA. Large choroidal vessels can appear congested, and leakage through the choriocapillaris and choroidal vessels results in a fuzzy appearance in late phases of ICGA (Fig. 24). Reduced-fluence photodynamic therapy covering the entire area

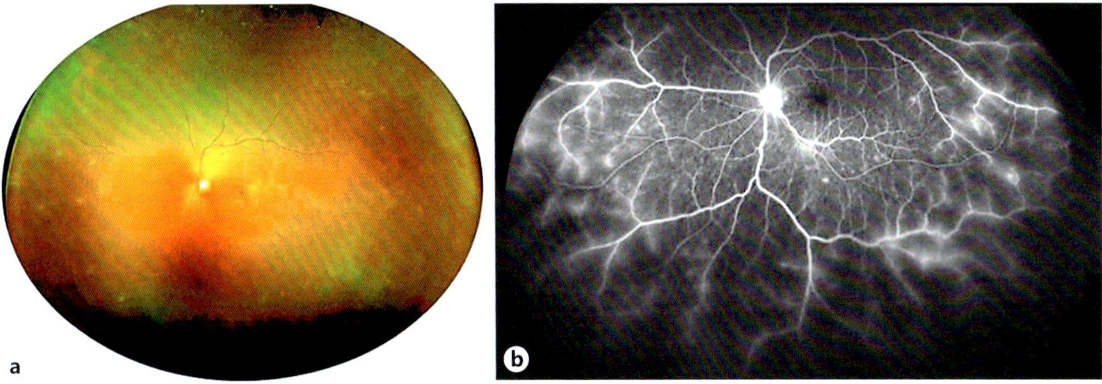

Fig. 28. Behçet's disease. The ultrawide-field color photograph is hazy due to vitritis. However, sheathing of peripheral vessels and small areas of retinitis can be seen (**a**). Fluorescein angiogram (**b**) shows extensive peripheral retinal vascular leakage and disc hyperfluorescence.

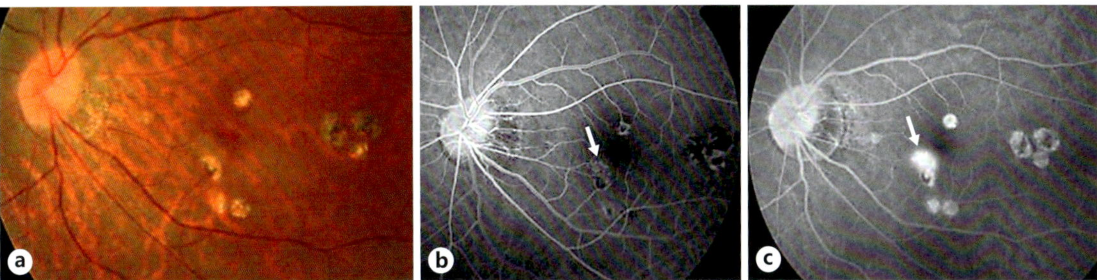

Fig. 29. Punctate inner choroidopathy complicated by secondary choroidal neovascularization (CNV). Multiple punctate lesions can be seen on the color fundus photograph (**a**). These lesions appear as window defects but do not leak on the fluorescein angiogram (**b**, **c**). In contrast, profuse leakage can be seen from a secondary active CNV (arrow).

of choroidal vascular hyperpermeability has been suggested to reduce the recurrence rate of CSC.

Chorioretinal Inflammatory Diseases

ICGA is useful to evaluate choroidal perfusion in choroidal inflammatory disease. Dark dots may appear on ICGA which may represent choroidal granuloma, choroidal nonperfusion, or even infarcts. Some examples of inflammatory conditions in which ICGA is useful include multiple evanescent white dot syndrome (Fig. 26), Vogt-Koyanagi-Harada disease (Fig. 27) [15], multifocal choroiditis, Behçet's disease (Fig. 28), acute multifocal posterior placoid pigment epitheliopathy [16], and ocular histoplasmosis syndrome. Secondary CNV may develop as a complication of inflammation. FA can help to differentiate active CNV from chorioretinal granuloma or RPE scars (Fig. 29).

Choroidal Tumors

ICGA is also indicated in the examination of choroidal tumors (Fig. 30). In melanomas, there may be corkscrew vessels seen within the lesion

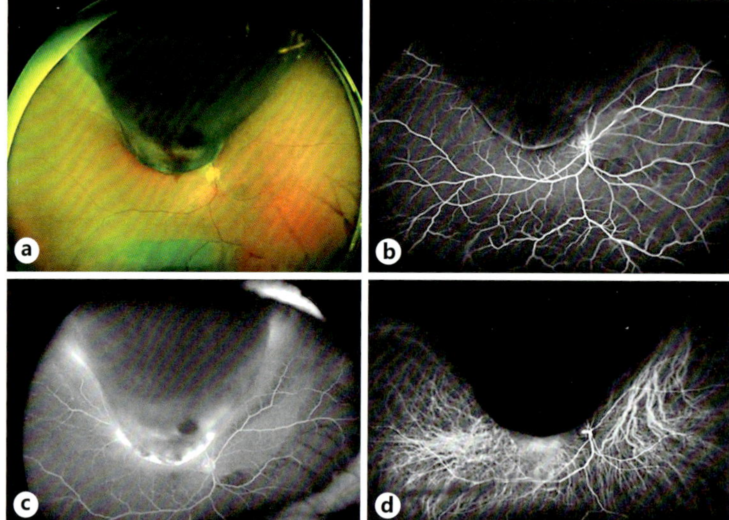

Fig. 30. Choroidal melanoma. A large elevated pigmented lesion can be seen in the superior retina extending to the fovea (**a**). Blocked fluorescence was seen within the lesion on the fluorescein angiogram (**b**, **c**) and indocyanine green angiogram (**d**).

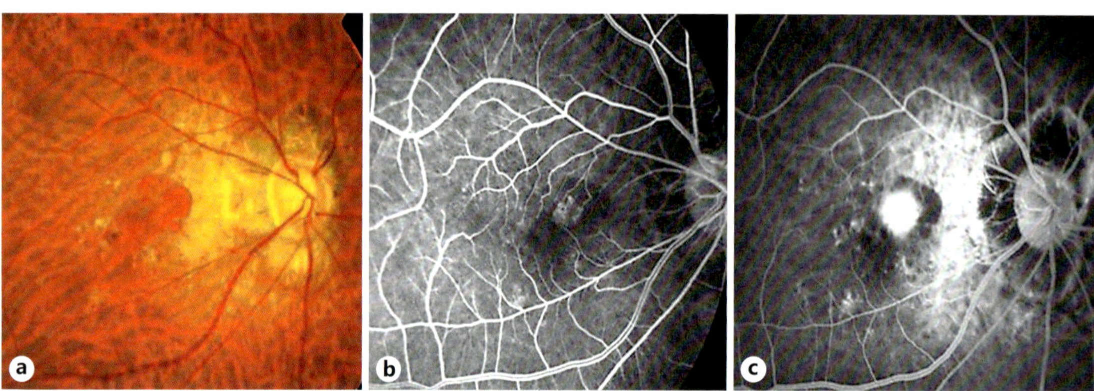

Fig. 31. Pathologic myopia with choroidal neovascularization. Features suggestive of pathologic myopia include tessellated fundus, yellowish appearance of diffuse chorioretinal atrophy in the posterior pole, as well as large peripapillary atrophy (**a**). On the fluorescein angiogram, an active juxtafoveal choroidal neovascularization with classic pattern can be seen (**b**, **c**).

on ICGA. In choroidal hemangioma, there is marked early hyperfluorescence with leakage and late staining on ICGA. Some lesions will have a speckled pattern within the lesion. In choroidal osteoma, small vessels are seen in the early phases of ICGA, but in the later phases there is diffuse hyperfluorescence, as well as some blocked fluorescence in the bony areas of the osteoma.

Pathologic Myopia and Myopic CNV

FA is considered the gold standard to confirm the diagnosis of CNV secondary to pathologic myopia (mCNV) [17–19]. mCNV typically appear as type 2 CNVs, with a classic leakage pattern (Fig. 31). Compared to neovascular AMD, there is usually less subretinal fluid or exudative changes associated with mCNV. Similarly, FA has been shown to be more sensitive than OCT in detecting activity in mCNV. mCNV can often be detected in close proximity to lacquer cracks. These are linear breaks in Bruch's membrane. Detection of lacquer cracks with conventional examination can be difficult. ICGA is widely accepted as the best method for detecting lacquer cracks, which typically appear as linear hypofluorescence in the late phase. When lacquer cracks develop or extend, subretinal hemorrhage may develop. These can be difficult to distinguish from mCNV on fundus examination, but can be readily differentiated based on FA and ICGA. In less severe stages of myopic maculopathy, diffuse atrophy is characterized by mild hyperfluorescence in late-phase FA and decrease in choroidal vasculature on ICGA. Areas of patchy chorioretinal atrophy are characterized by well-defined areas of hypofluorescence on FA and ICGA due to choroidal filling defect.

Conclusion

Fundus photography is a noninvasive imaging modality that can document fundus signs, and is useful for screening program, as well as in conjunction with other imaging modalities for evaluation of more complex diseases. FA and ICGA provide information on the retinal as well as choroidal circulation, and indirectly the status of the RPE. This information is useful in the diagnosis and treatment planning of many conditions which have been covered in this chapter. With advances in technology, these imaging modalities will provide complementary information to other newer imaging technologies, such as OCT.

References

1 Grading diabetic retinopathy from stereoscopic color fundus photographs – an extension of the modified Airlie House classification. ETDRS report number 10. Early Treatment Diabetic Retinopathy Study Research Group. Ophthalmology 1991;98(suppl):786–806.

2 Wong TY, Cheung CM, Larsen M, Sharma S, Simo R: Diabetic retinopathy. Nat Rev Dis Primers 2016;2:16012.

3 Klein R, Davis MD, Magli YL, Segal P, Klein BE, Hubbard L: The Wisconsin age-related maculopathy grading system. Ophthalmology 1991;98:1128–1134.

4 Wong WL, Su X, Li X, Cheung CM, Klein R, Cheng CY, Wong TY: Global prevalence of age-related macular degeneration and disease burden projection for 2020 and 2040: a systematic review and meta-analysis. Lancet Glob Health 2014;2:e106–e116.

5 Age-Related Eye Disease Study Research Group: A randomized, placebo-controlled, clinical trial of high-dose supplementation with vitamins C and E and beta carotene for age-related cataract and vision loss: AREDS report No. 9. Arch Ophthalmol 2001;119:1439–1452.

6 Vitale S, Clemons TE, Agron E, Ferris FL 3rd, Domalpally A, Danis RP, Chew EY; Age-Related Eye Disease Study 2 Research Group: Evaluating the validity of the Age-Related Eye Disease Study Grading Scale for age-related macular degeneration: AREDS2 Report 10. JAMA Ophthalmol 2016;134:1041–1047.

7 Silva PS, Cavallerano JD, Sun JK, Soliman AZ, Aiello LM, Aiello LP: Peripheral lesions identified by mydriatic ultrawide field imaging: distribution and potential impact on diabetic retinopathy severity. Ophthalmology 2013;120:2587–2595.

8 Silva PS, Cavallerano JD, Tolls D, Omar A, Thakore K, Patel B, Sehizadeh M, Tolson AM, Sun JK, Aiello LM, et al: Potential efficiency benefits of nonmydriatic ultrawide field retinal imaging in an ocular telehealth diabetic retinopathy program. Diabetes Care 2014;37:50–55.

9 Tsai ASH, Cheung N, Gan ATL, Jaffe GJ, Sivaprasad S, Wong TY, Cheung CMG: Retinal angiomatous proliferation. Surv Ophthalmol 2017;62:462–492.

10 Wong CW, Wong TY, Cheung CM: Polypoidal choroidal vasculopathy in Asians. J Clin Med 2015;4:782–821.

11 Wong CW, Yanagi Y, Lee WK, Ogura Y, Yeo I, Wong TY, Cheung CMG: Age-related macular degeneration and polypoidal choroidal vasculopathy in Asians. Prog Retin Eye Res 2016;53:107–139.

12 Cheung CM, Lai TY, Chen SJ, Chong V, Lee WK, Htoon H, Ng WY, Ogura Y, Wong TY: Understanding indocyanine green angiography in polypoidal choroidal vasculopathy: the group experience with digital fundus photography and confocal scanning laser ophthalmoscopy. Retina 2014;34:2397–2406.

13 Cheung CM, Laude A, Wong W, Mathur R, Chan CM, Wong E, Wong D, Wong TY, Lim TH: Improved specificity of polypoidal choroidal vasculopathy diagnosis using a modified Everest criteria. Retina 2015;35:1375–1380.

14 Tan GS, Cheung N, Simo R, Cheung GC, Wong TY: Diabetic macular oedema. Lancet Diabetes Endocrinol 2017;5:143–155.

15 Chee SP, Jap A, Cheung CM: The prognostic value of angiography in Vogt-Koyanagi-Harada disease. Am J Ophthalmol 2010;150:888–893.

16 Cheung CM, Yeo IY, Koh A: Photoreceptor changes in acute and resolved acute posterior multifocal placoid pigment epitheliopathy documented by spectral-domain optical coherence tomography. Arch Ophthalmol 2010;128:644–646.

17 Ohno-Matsui K, Lai TY, Lai CC, Cheung CM: Updates of pathologic myopia. Prog Retin Eye Res 2016;52:156–187.

18 Cheung CMG, Arnold JJ, Holz FG, Park KH, Lai TYY, Larsen M, Mitchell P, Ohno-Matsui K, Chen SJ, Wolf S, et al: Myopic choroidal neovascularization: review, guidance, and consensus statement on management. Ophthalmology 2017;124:1690–1711.

19 Neelam K, Cheung CM, Ohno-Matsui K, Lai TY, Wong TY: Choroidal neovascularization in pathological myopia. Prog Retin Eye Res 2012;31:495–525.

Assoc. Prof. Gemmy C.M. Cheung
Singapore National Eye Center
11 Third Hospital Avenue
Singapore (Singapore)
E-Mail gemmy.cheung.c.m@singhealth.com.sg

Cheung · Koh

Cunha-Vaz J, Koh A (eds): Imaging Techniques.
ESASO Course Series. Basel, Karger, 2018, vol 10, pp 19–36 (DOI: 10.1159/000487410)

Optical Coherence Tomography: Retinal Imaging

Colin S. Tan[a, b] · Wei Kiong Ngo[a] · Srinivas R. Sadda[c]

[a]National Healthcare Group Eye Institute, Tan Tock Seng Hospital, and [b]Fundus Image Reading Center, National Healthcare Group Eye Institute, Singapore, Singapore; [c]Doheny Eye Institute, University of California Los Angeles, Los Angeles, CA, USA

Abstract

Optical coherence tomography (OCT) is a noninvasive investigation that produces detailed, high-resolution images of ocular structures in both the anterior and posterior segments of the eye. OCT is used to assess the retina quantitatively and qualitatively, and these parameters have been used both in clinical practice and as outcome measures in multicenter randomized controlled clinical trials. The features identified on OCT are used for the diagnosis, monitoring of disease activity, and assessing response to treatment. Quantitative features measured using OCT include retinal thickness and volumes, and choroidal thickness. OCT can also detect features of disease activity, such as retinal thickening, intraretinal cysts, subretinal fluid, and choroidal neovascular membranes located in the subretinal and sub-retinal pigment epithelial space. In addition, OCT can provide structural information of the normal anatomy and pathological features seen in many retinal conditions. OCT has proven invaluable in the diagnosis and monitoring of diseases such as age-related macular degeneration, polypoidal choroidal vasculopathy, diabetic retinopathy, retinal vein occlusions, and pathological myopia. This chapter provides an evidence-based review on the features of some of these common retinal conditions, and discusses the application of OCT in their assessment and management.

© 2018 S. Karger AG, Basel

Since the introduction of optical coherence tomography (OCT) two decades ago [1], this technology has revolutionized the practice of ophthalmology as well as other branches of medicine. OCT produces noninvasive, high-resolution images of both the anterior segment (cornea and structures at the angles) and posterior segment (retina, choroid, sclera, and optic disc) of the eye (Fig. 1).

OCT is based on the principle of low-coherence interferometry. Using an optical source to

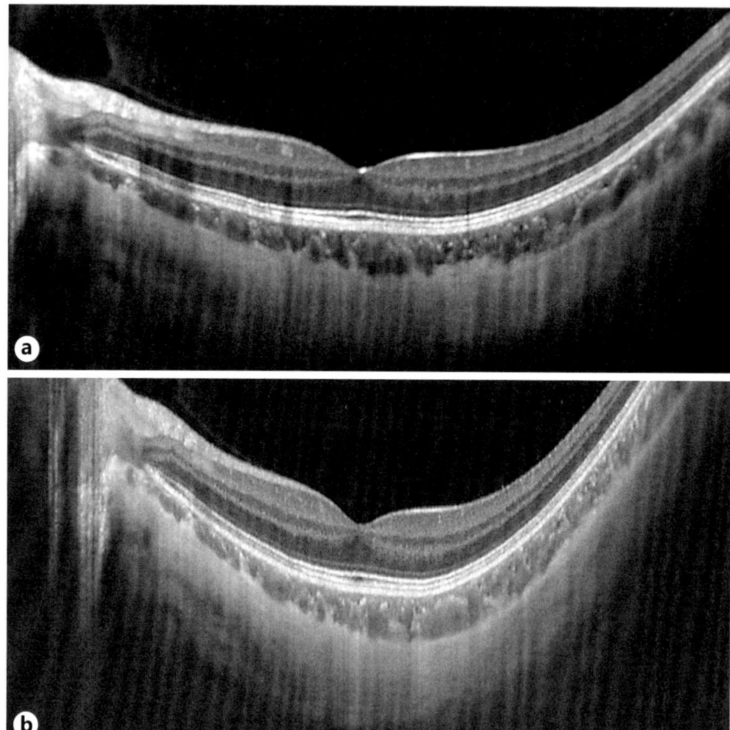

Fig. 1. Optical coherence tomography (OCT) scan of a normal eye. **a** Spectral-domain OCT scan. **b** Swept source OCT scan of the same eye.

direct a low-coherence light beam at a surface, an interferometer detects the reflected optical data and reads the data as an interference pattern to create a depth profile (known as an A-scan). Multiple scans along the sample in a linear fashion create a cross-sectional image (B-scan). Combining multiple B-scans enables a three-dimensional volume scan of the tissue. Current technology allows for micron-scale imaging of tissue microstructure, while the penetration depth of each scan is in the order of millimeters.

Evolution of OCT

Earlier time-domain OCT machines used low-coherence light from a superluminescent diode and mechanically translated a reference mirror axially to build up a depth image. Scanning mirrors were then used to scan the region of interest at various locations. Therefore, time-domain OCT was limited by the speed at which the reference mirror could be moved. A-scans rates on time-domain OCT devices were limited to 400 A-scans per second.

The next evolution of OCT, spectral-domain OCT (SD-OCT) had no moving reference mirrors. Instead, light from a superluminescent diode light source was used together with a fixed reference mirror to generate a broadband interference pattern. This interference pattern was then detected with spectrally separated detectors. Either a superluminescent diode or femtosecond laser was used as the broadband source, but a spectrometer was used instead of a photodetector. The early SD-OCT devices produced between 20,000 and 40,000 A-scans per second, while current SD-OCT devices can scan at 70,000 A-scans per second.

Swept-source domain OCT (SS-OCT) is the latest generation of OCT (Fig. 1b). It utilizes a tunable source laser that rapidly sweeps across a broad bandwidth, typically centered on 1,050 nm [2, 3]. SS-OCT converts the signal from spectral interferometry to a depth profile using Fourier transformation of the interference pattern. The advantages of this technology are that it is more sensitive (theoretically 20–30 dB better) than time-domain OCT and is able to scan 100–1,000 times faster than time-domain OCT.

Assessment of Retinal Conditions Using OCT

OCT can be used to assess retinal conditions both quantitatively and qualitatively. The qualitative features seen on OCT will be discussed in subsequent sections in relation to specific clinical conditions.

Quantitatively, retinal thickness and volume can be measured using OCT. These have been used in clinical practice and multicenter randomized controlled clinical trials to determine disease activity and response to treatment. It is important, however, to note that retinal thickness measurements made using different OCT devices are not comparable, especially between time-domain OCT and spectral-domain OCT [4–6]. This is the result of differences in location of the segmentation boundaries that are used to determine retinal thickness [4–6].

When assessing retinal thickness, it is important to consider potential ocular and demographic factors that may affect this. Central subfield macular thickness does not vary significantly with refractive error [7–9]. In contrast, the peripheral retina thins progressively with increasing myopia [10, 11], and this needs to be taken into consideration if retinal thickness in this region is being assessed. Also important to consider is the potential impact of diurnal variation in thickness measurements during the day. While retinal thickness does not vary significantly at different times of the day, studies have demonstrated that the choroid exhibits a distinct diurnal variation [12].

Applications of OCT to Various Retinal Conditions

Age-Related Macular Degeneration

Age-related macular degeneration (AMD) is the most common cause of visual impairment in developed countries. Its prevalence is expected to increase as a result of the ageing population trends observed in many parts of the world. OCT is integral to the diagnosis and monitoring of AMD both in clinical practice and multicenter randomized controlled trials. In addition to confirming the diagnosis of AMD, it can be used to subtype the choroidal neovascularization (CNV) lesion and to determine disease activity.

The earliest sign of AMD is the presence of drusen (Fig. 2). Histopathologically, drusen are located between the retinal pigment epithelium (RPE) and Bruch membrane (BM) and represents accumulations of hydrophobic extracellular material. Larger drusen may appear on OCT as a hyperreflective separation of the RPE and BM, known as a drusenoid PED (pigment epithelial detachment) [13] (Fig. 3).

Reticular pseudodrusen was first described by Mimoun et al. [14] using blue light reflectance imaging. Recently, there has been much interest in reticular pseudodrusen as a marker predicting development of choroidal neovascularization in AMD [15]. On OCT, these lesions are shown as granular hyperreflective deposits situated between the RPE layer and the ellipsoid zone that raises the ellipsoid zone into an undulating layer [16] (Fig. 4). Arnold et al. [15] also found that reticular pseudodrusen was associated with significant choroidal thinning.

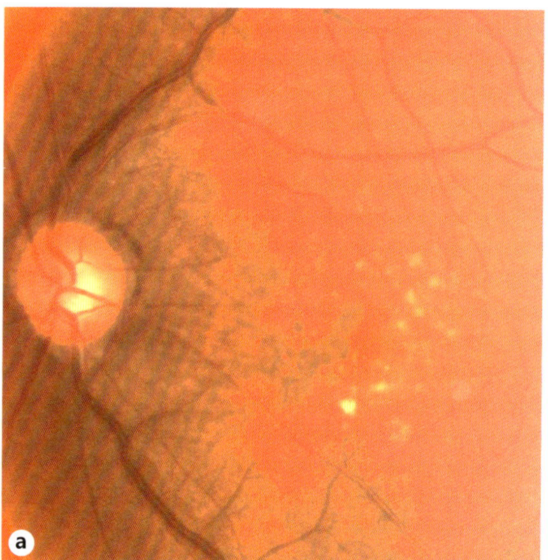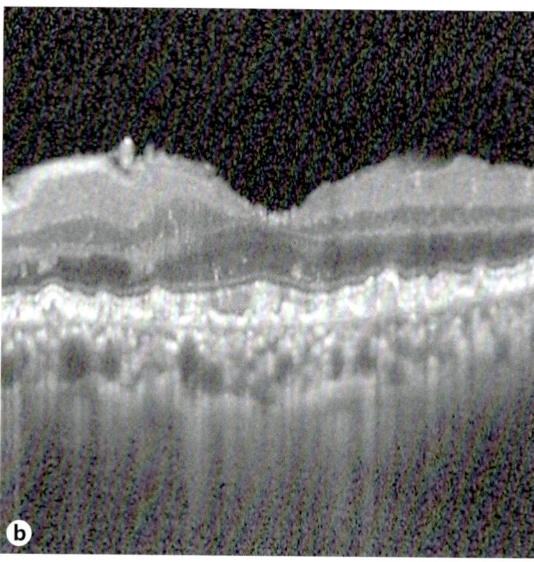

Fig. 2. Non-neovascular age-related macular degeneration. **a** Color fundus photograph showing drusen. **b** Optical coherence tomography scan illustrating multiple small drusen located beneath the retinal pigment epithelium.

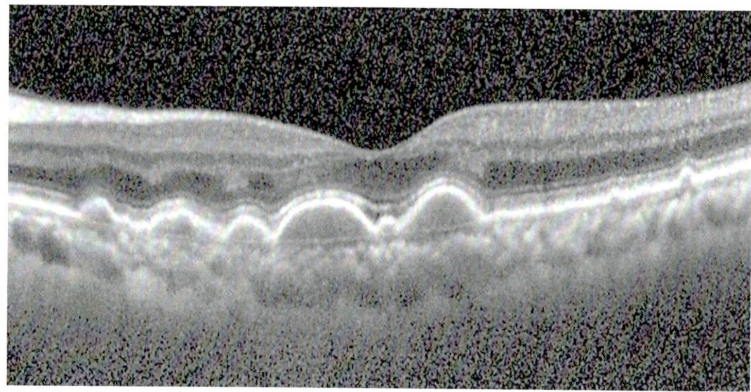

Fig. 3. Drusenoid pigment epithelial detachment. These are characterized by smooth elevations of the retinal pigment epithelium (RPE) and a homogenous appearance beneath the RPE.

Among eyes with neovascular AMD, OCT is used to visualize the macular NV lesion, which has been classified into several types:

1 Type 1 CNV. In this type, the CNV lesion is located beneath the RPE, often under an elevation of the RPE. It appears as highly reflective fibrovascular tissue with irregular yet defined borders [17] (Fig. 5a). On fluorescein angiography (FA), type 1 CNV usually manifests with an occult pattern of leakage (Fig. 5b–d).

2 Type 2 CNV. The CNV lesion is located in the subretinal space, between the ellipsoid zone and RPE. The lesion has breached the RPE, causing focal disruption of the RPE (Fig. 6). This usually appears as classic CNV on FA.

3 Type 3 NV. More recently, type 3 neovascularization has been described, and is associated with retinal angiomatous proliferation. Type 3 NV originates within the deep neural retina, and consists of a

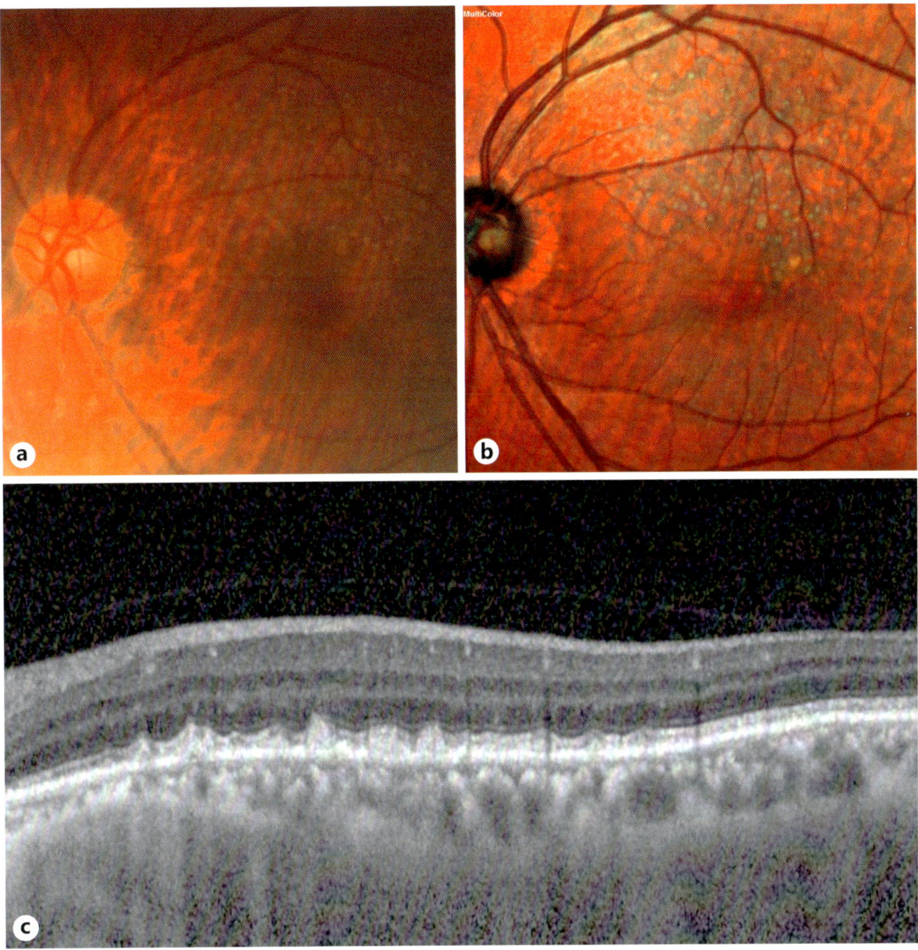

Fig. 4. Reticular pseudodrusen. **a** Color fundus photograph illustrating the reticular pseudodrusen as fine granular lesions superior to the fovea. **b** Multicolor imaging using the Heidelberg Spectralis device. The reticular pseudodrusen appear more distinct on the multicolor image. **c** Optical coherence tomography scan. The reticular pseudodrusen appear between the ellipsoid zone and the retinal pigment epithelium.

hyperreflective, linear lesion. These lesions can eventually extend to involve the subretinal and/or sub-RPE spaces.

In addition to visualization of the NV lesion, the features of disease activity in neovascular AMD include:

1 Subretinal fluid
2 Intraretinal cysts
3 Retinal thickening and edema
4 Retinal PEDs
5 RPE tears or rips. These usually occur at the edge of a PED
6 Subretinal or sub-RPE scars. These appear as hyperreflective regions within the subretinal space or beneath the RPE, and are an indication of chronic disease.

Polypoidal Choroidal Vasculopathy
Polypoidal choroidal vasculopathy (PCV) was first described by Yannuzzi et al. [18] in 1990,

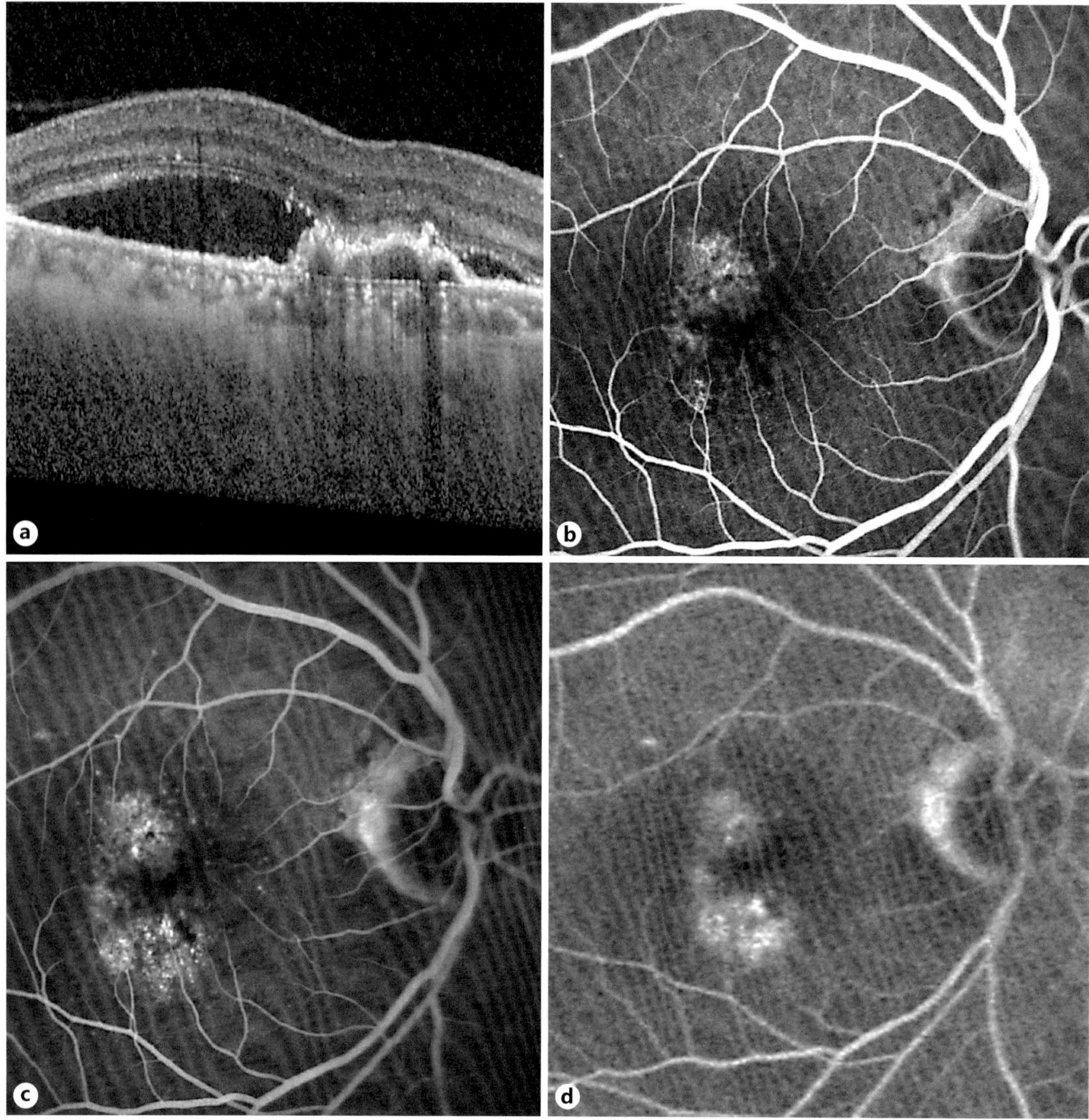

Fig. 5. Type 1 choroidal neovascularization. **a** The optical coherence tomography (OCT) scan shows elevation of the retinal pigment epithelium, with hyperreflectivity beneath this. There is also subretinal fluid. The choroid is also clearly visualized on this OCT scan. **b** Early phase of the fluorescein angiogram (FA). **c** Midphase of the FA showing stippled hyperfluorescence. **d** Late phase of the FA showing slight increase in leakage.

who termed it idiopathic PCV at that time. PCV is a variant of exudative AMD [19] and consists of abnormal vascular network and terminal dilatations which form the polyps. Among patients with neovascular AMD, its prevalence varies among different populations, but it has been described to occur in 25–55% of Asian patients with neovascular AMD [20]. The gold standard for diagnosis of PCV is indocyanine green angiography (ICGA) [21] (Fig. 7a, b). While different diagnos-

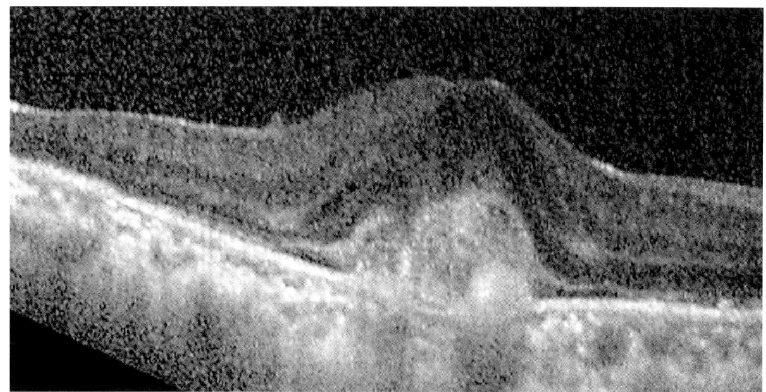

Fig. 6. Type 2 choroidal neovascularization (CNV). Optical coherence tomography demonstrating subretinal hyperreflectivity corresponding to the type 2 CNV lesion.

tic criteria have been described, a robust and commonly used diagnostic criterion has been utilized in the EVEREST and EVEREST II studies [21–25]. OCT, on the other hand, is an important adjunct in the diagnosis and monitoring of the disease.

On OCT, the lesion components in PCV have the following appearances:

1 A focal, sharp/tented elevation of the RPE. This is in contrast to a typical PED, which has a broader base, and smoother elevation [26, 27].
2 A roundish lesion with hyperreflective borders and hyporeflective center which is located beneath the RPE elevation. This is believed to be the actual polyp [26–28] (Fig. 7c).
3 An additional elevation of the RPE which frequently occurs at the edge of the larger PED. This is known as the "double-hump sign," and is usually the location of a polyp [26, 27].
4 Two separate hyperreflective lines at the level of the RPE, known as the "double-layer" sign. This is believed to correspond to the location of the branching vascular network [29–32] (Fig. 7d).

The indications of disease activity in PCV that are seen on OCT are similar to Type 1 CNV. Patients often manifest with subretinal fluid and PEDs. There may also be hyperreflectivity in the

subretinal space corresponding to subretinal hemorrhage. Among patients with PCV, increased frequency of serous retinal detachments (RD) (78% in PCV vs. 53% in AMD), increased height of the serous RD (56.3 μm in PCV vs. 21.9 μm in AMD), and less intraretinal fluid and cysts are seen compared with neovascular AMD [31, 33].

On EDI-OCT, the choroid appears thicker in eyes with PCV compared to normal controls or eyes with AMD [34]. Recently, PCV has been described to be one disease entity among the pachychoroid spectrum of diseases.

In a study of 17 eyes with PCV observed using SD-OCT, the authors found that all 17 eyes showed subretinal fluid (serous RD) in association with PEDs. SD-OCT scans passing through the PCV complex identified on ICGA showed that all had a sub-RPE hyperreflective tissue similar to what is seen in type 1 (occult) CNV. None of the eyes showed evidence of type 2 CNV. All eyes had PEDs that were atypical in morphology and content. They assumed a corrugated or "bumpy" configuration. In some of the cases, the bumps of the RPE line were markedly abrupt, yielding an "M-shaped" or even a "QRS complex-shaped" PED. Careful analysis of the contents of these PEDs yielded well-delineated, round to oval, sub-RPE cavities with low to medium reflectivity centrally, and hyperreflective borders resembling vascular cavities

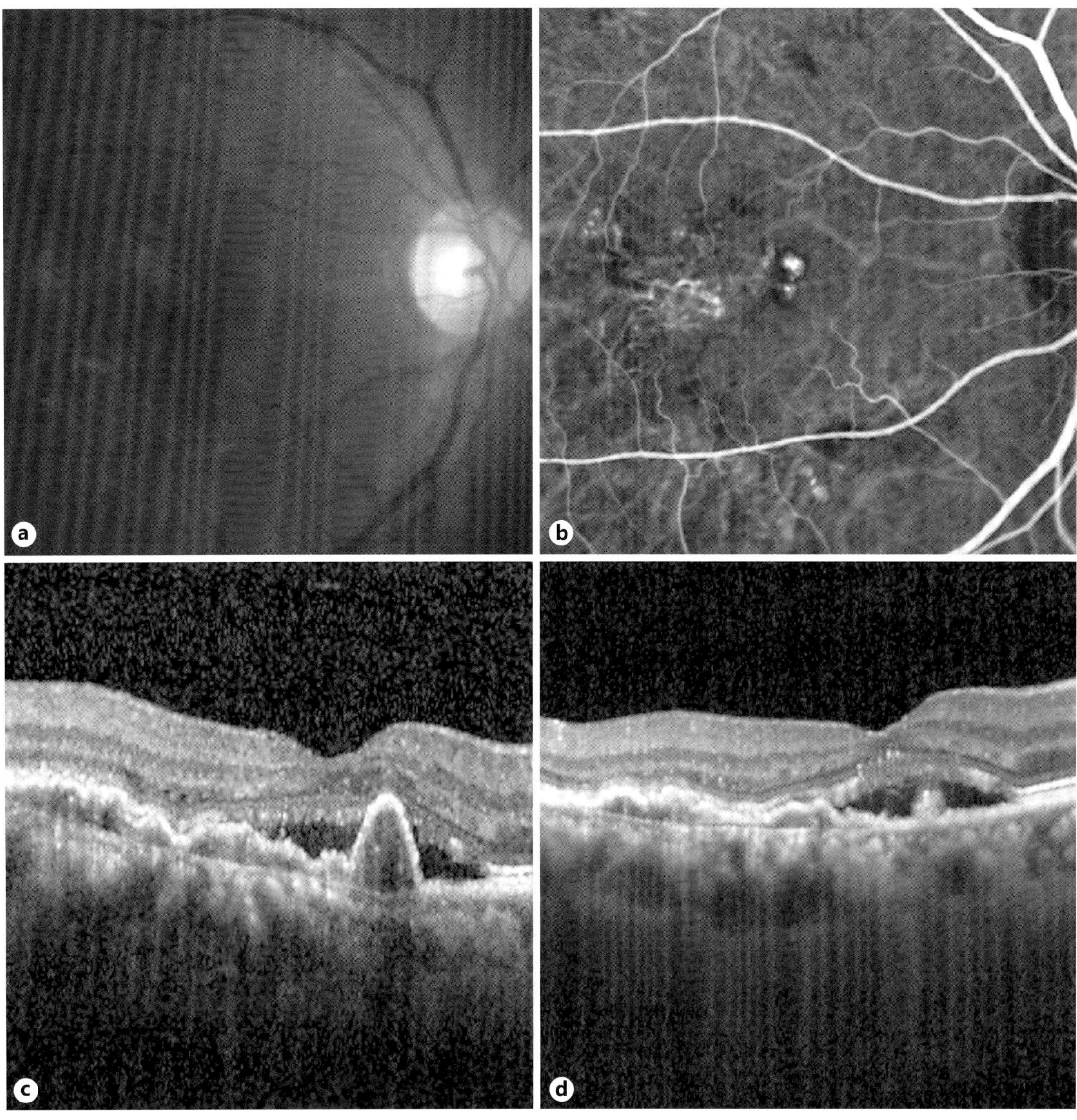

Fig. 7. Polypoidal choroidal vasculopathy (PCV). **a** Color fundus photograph showing an orange-red subretinal nodule. **b** Indocyanine green angiogram showing the PCV lesion, which consists of the polyps and a branching vascular network (BVN). **c** Optical coherence tomography (OCT) scan through one of the polyps, showing a sharp elevation of the retinal pigment epithelium (RPE). There is subretinal fluid surrounding the RPE elevation. **d** OCT scan through the BVN, showing undulation of the RPE, which is sometimes referred to as a "double-layer sign."

[35]. Sa et al. [28] also suggested that this attenuation of internal reflectivity within the PED on OCT images strongly supported PCV diagnosis with a sensitivity of 84% and a specificity of 94%.

In a study by De Salvo et al. [27], the authors reviewed SD-OCTs of 51 eyes with 1 or more PEDs attributable to either PCV or occult CNV based on qualitative features such as sharp PED peak, PED notch, and hyporeflective lumen with-

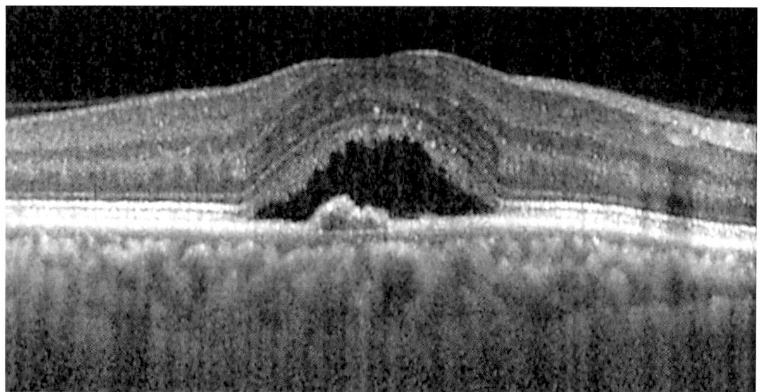

Fig. 8. Central serous chorioretinopathy. Optical coherence tomography scan showing subretinal fluid with elongation of the photoreceptor outer segments. There is also elevation of the retinal pigment epithelium, corresponding to the area of leakage.

in hyperreflective lesions adherent to RPE to make a final diagnosis of PCV. When compared to the diagnosis made on ICGA and FA, OCT detected 35 of 37 true-positive PCV lesions but missed 2 ICGA-confirmed lesions (false negatives). Also, OCT excluded 13 of 14 non-PCV lesions but misidentified 1 PCV lesion (false positive). These data showed a sensitivity of 94.6% and a specificity of 92.9% for using OCT to diagnose PCV [27].

Central Serous Chorioretinopathy

Central serous chorioretinopathy (CSCR) is a maculopathy characterized by a smooth serous RD with subretinal fluid (Fig. 8). It is often idiopathic, although it may be associated with chronic steroid use or stress.

On OCT, the characteristics of CSCR are as follows:

1. Smooth elevation of the neuorosensory retina, associated with subretinal fluid (Fig. 8).

2. Sometimes, an elevation of the RPE or small PED may be observed. These often correspond to the areas of leakage seen on FA or ICGA.

3. Elongation of the photoreceptor outer segments, especially among eyes with a longer duration of disease [36, 37].

4. Thickening of the choroid, with enlargement of the choroidal vessels [38].

In a study of 21 eyes, RPE abnormalities were observed in 96% of eyes with acute CSCR, with a minute defect of the RPE occurring within the PED. This appeared to correspond precisely to the leakage point seen on FA in 5 eyes (22%) [37].

The microstructural morphology of the detached retina also showed interesting findings. When the retina detached, the appearance of the outer retinal layer changed; the external limiting membrane persisted, although the ellipsoid zone could not be detected in all eyes [39]. In the acute phase, the thickness of the probable photoreceptor outer segment increased in the entire area of the detached retina. The increased thickness of the photoreceptor outer segment in the detached retina decreased gradually, and the outer segment's appearance changed to granular until reattachment of the retina [39].

Diabetic Retinopathy

Among patients with diabetic macular edema (DME), the features typically seen on OCT (Fig. 9a) include:

1   Diffuse retinal thickening. This is described as generalized, heterogeneous, mild hyporeflectivity compared with normal retina with an elevated mean central subfield thickness compared to the normative value for that OCT device. It is a feature reported to be present in at least 88% of eyes with DME [40–42].

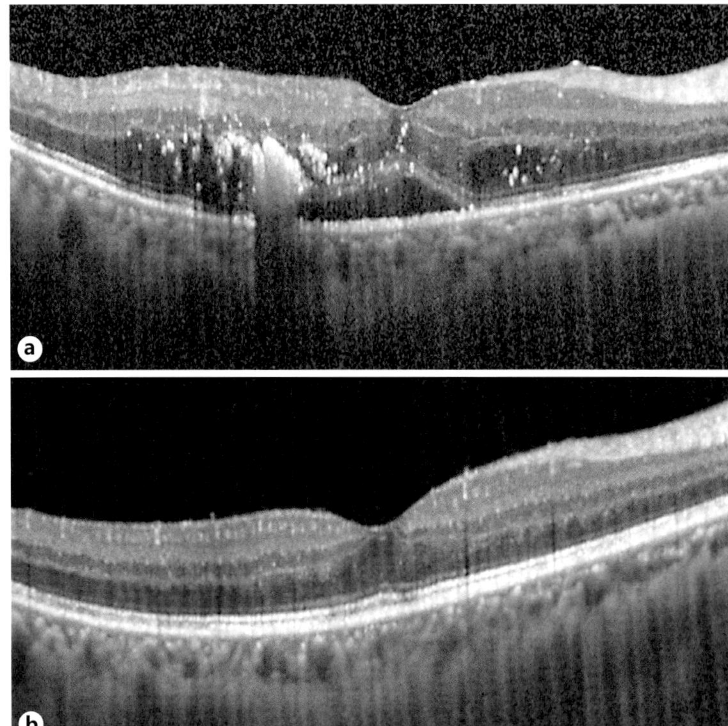

Fig. 9. Diabetic macular edema. **a** Optical coherence tomography (OCT) scan showing retinal thickening and intraretinal cysts. An area of hyperreflectivity corresponds to hard exudates. There is also subretinal fluid. **b** OCT scan of the same eye showing resolution of the edema and hard exudates following treatment with anti-VEGF agents.

2 Cystoid macular edema is identified as the presence of round or oval intraretinal cystoid areas of hyporeflectivity, typically separated by hyperreflective septae. It is typically present in 44–47% of eyes with DME [40–42].

3 Serous RD. The prevalence of subfoveal serous RD has been reported in 3–31% of patients with DME [41, 43–45].

4 Hard exudates. These consist of lipoproteins that are deposited in the outer plexiform layer of the retina, and appear as hyperreflective nodular or small lesions in the outer plexiform layer on OCT (Fig. 9).

5 Cotton wool spots are ischemic infarctions of the nerve fiber layer and appear as hyperreflective, nodular, or elongated lesions in the nerve fiber layer on OCT.

6 Hemorrhages are hyperreflective on OCT and can produce shadowing on the outer retinal layers [46].

7 Vitreomacular traction (VMT). These appear as hyperreflective bands that are attached to the internal limiting membrane at specific sites and are usually sharply elevated. In some cases, they exert traction on the retina, and result in distortion of the retinal anatomy.

8 Epiretinal membrane. Epiretinal membrane is seen as a hyperreflective band along the inner aspect of the inner limiting membrane.

The pathophysiology of macular edema has been linked to VMT [47]. In cases of persistent DME, vitreomacular interface abnormalities such as VMT and epiretinal membrane formation were found to be highly prevalent. Therefore, in macular edema cases with traction, vitrectomy to release a taut adherent posterior hyaloid is the treatment of choice as traditional laser photocoagulation was found to be ineffective [47–50]. Some patients do not

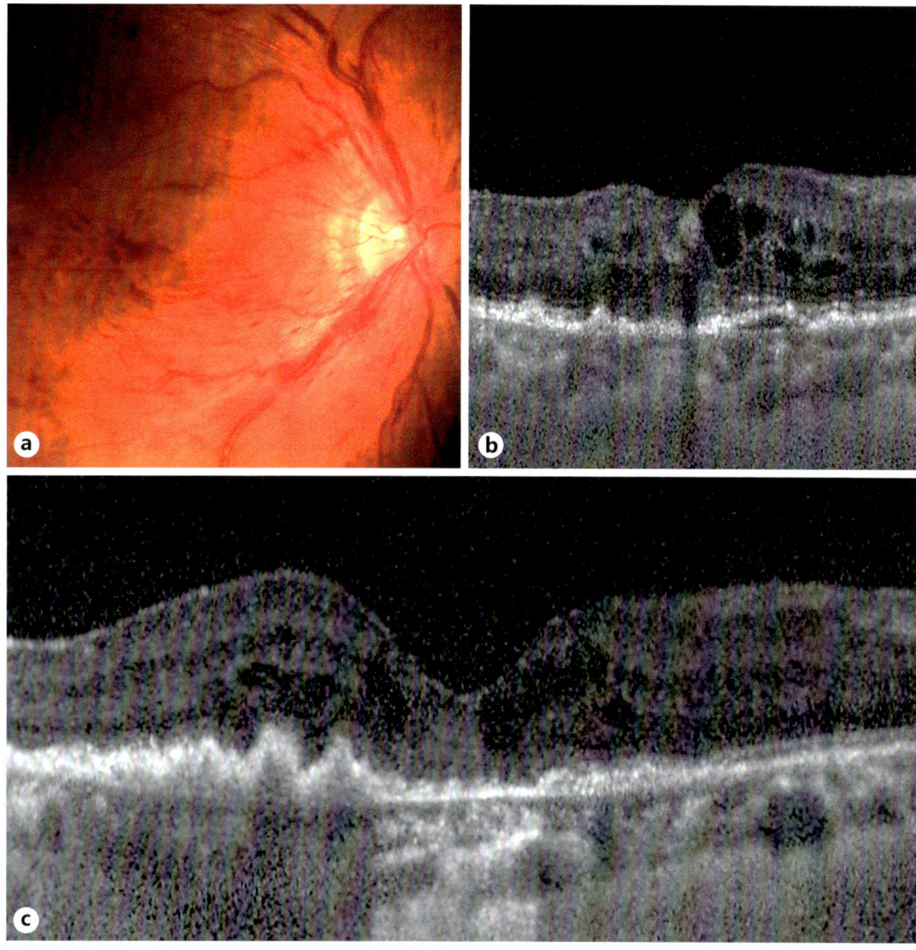

Fig. 10. Central retinal vein occlusion. **a** Color fundus photograph showing flame and blot hemorrhages, together with venous tortuosity. **b** Optical coherence tomography (OCT) scan through the fovea showing retinal thickening and intraretinal cysts. **c** OCT scan through the same region following treatment with anti-VEGF agents. Although the retinal thickening has reduced, there is persistent cystoid macular edema. In addition, there is photoreceptor atrophy centrally, with increased transmission of signal beneath this.

regain vision despite reduction in retinal thickening after treatment. This may be related to the integrity of foveal photoreceptors. Disruption of the ellipsoid zone has been reported to occur in 49–75% of patients with DME [40, 51, 52]. Greater visual improvement was observed in those with an intact ellipsoid zone following successful treatment [40] (Fig. 9b).

Retinal Vein Occlusion

Patients with retinal vein occlusion (Fig. 10a) may develop macular edema, which is currently treated with anti-VEGF therapy. Many of the features of retinal vein occlusion are similar to those seen in DME, as described above. These include diffuse retinal thickening, cystoid macular edema, and subretinal fluid (Fig. 10b).

In addition, the following features may be seen in patients with retinal vein occlusion:

1 Retinal hemorrhages in retinal vein occlusions are detected as corresponding amorphous and moderately hyperreflective lesions located in both the inner retina (flame-shaped hemorrhages) and outer retina (blot hemorrhages), often extending to the outer plexiform layer [53].
2 Prominent middle-limiting membrane sign is seen as a hyperreflective line at the inner synaptic portion of the outer plexiform layer. It occurs in 28% of cases and is associated with ischemic central retinal vein occlusion [54].
3 Paracentral acute middle maculopathy (PAMM) manifests as hyperreflectivity within the inner nuclear layer seen on OCT. It is a variant of acute macular neuroretinopathy. Vaso-occlusion results in deep retinal capillary ischemia, and this has been observed in RVO among other conditions [55].
4 After retinal vein occlusion, inner retinal atrophy is associated with poor visual acuity following the resolution of baseline macular edema [56]. The inner retinal layers appear thinner and less distinct compared to a normal OCT scan (Fig. 10c).

Retinal Artery Occlusion

In patients with retinal artery occlusion, OCT findings in the acute stage include increased reflectivity of all the inner retinal layers with diffuse parafoveolar thickening and decreased reflectivity from the perifoveolar RPE [57, 58] (Fig. 11).

Increased edema on OCT was associated with a smaller cherry-red spot. Intracellular edema may cause ganglion cell displacement toward the central fovea, subsequently obscuring the borders of the cherry-red spot, resulting in a smaller cherry-red spot on exam [59] (Fig. 11).

Several months after the acute episode of arterial occlusion, OCT scans manifest with increased thickness and hyperreflectivity of the inner retinal layers, followed by gradual reduction in retinal thickness and eventual atrophy of all retinal layers [60, 61].

PAMM is defined by hyperreflectivity in the middle retinal layers at the level of the inner nuclear layer on OCT. It has also been reported in RAO. Yu et al. [62] described a prevalence of 22% for PAMM amongst 40 eyes with RAO.

Myopia

Myopia is a common condition among some populations, especially among Asians [63–65]. High myopia is defined as a spherical equivalent of –6 dpt or higher. Patients with myopia often manifest with structural changes which can be detected using OCT (Fig. 12).

1. Posterior staphyloma. A posterior staphyloma is a limited area of outpouching of the posterior segment and represents a deformity of eyes with pathological myopia [66]. While the best method of detecting the presence of a staphyloma has not been determined, OCT is a useful tool to delineate the shape of the sclera to show the posterior bowing. Ohno-Matsui et al. [66] used swept-source OCT to determine the entire thickness of the sclera and the contour of the sclera in many highly myopic eyes. However, the scan length of current commercially available OCT instruments is not long enough to cover the entire extent of a wide staphyloma in some eyes.

2. Dome-shaped macula (DSM) (Fig. 13). A DSM exhibits a convex, curved, elevated profile of the posterior pole, sometimes within the concavity of the staphyloma [67]. While features of a DSM can be detected clinically, it is very clearly seen on OCT. The RPE manifest with a smooth, convex elevation at the macula, often with changes of the underlying choroid profile. The bulge may be associated with a local thickening of subfoveal sclera [68]. DSM is associated with visual impairment and metamorphopsia. Several com-

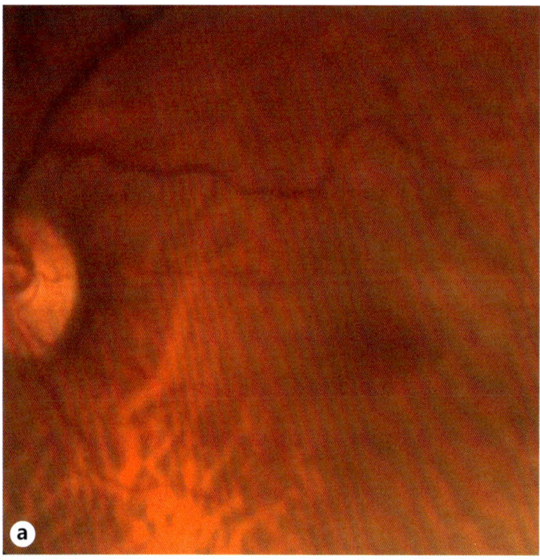

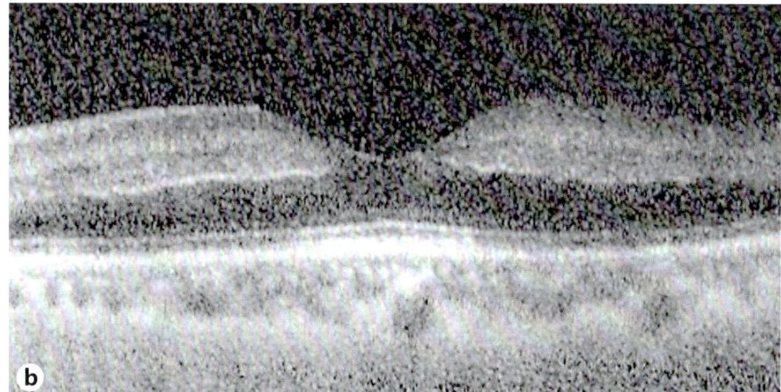

Fig. 11. Central retinal artery occlusion. **a** Color fundus photography showing a pale retina with a cherry-red spot. **b** Optical coherence tomography scan showing thickening and increased hyperreflectivity of the retinal layers.

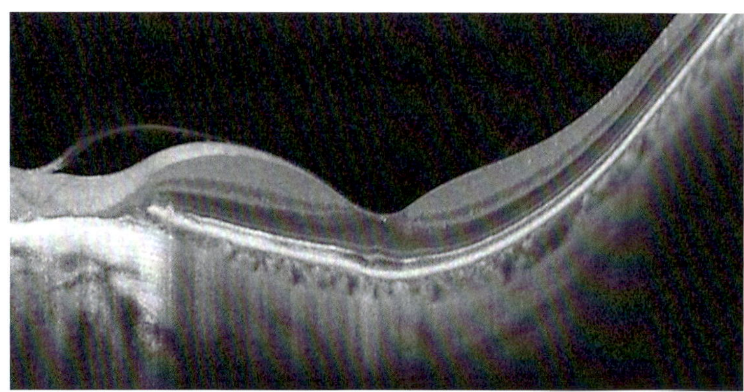

Fig. 12. High myopia. Optical coherence tomography scan showing increased curvature of the posterior pole, consistent with a staphyloma. There is increased peripapillary atrophy and thinning of the retina temporally. The choroid is also relatively thin.

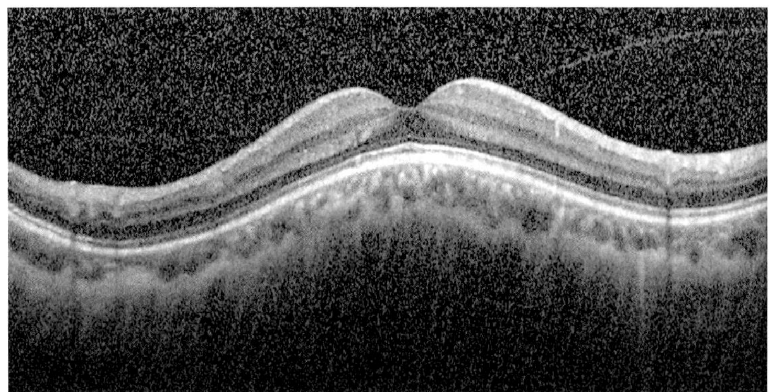

Fig. 13. Dome-shaped macula. There is a smooth elevation of the retinal pigment epithelium beneath the macula, giving a convex, dome-shaped appearance. The choroid is also elevated beneath the dome-shaped macula.

plications resulting in visual loss in DSM have been described, including atrophic changes in the RPE, foveal serous RD, and development of CNV. Complications among eyes with DSM were reported to be as high as 60.29%, and included CNV, subretinal fluid without CNV, atrophy, or macular hole [67, 69].

3. Myopic foveoschisis. Macular foveoschisis is more common in Asians and its prevalence ranges from 9 to 34%. On OCT, macular foveoschisis appears as a collection of intraretinal cyst separating the retina into an outer layer and an inner layer, with bridging columns that are hyperreflective [70].

4. Macular holes. Patients with myopia may also develop macular holes, which can be detected clinically. However, OCT is invaluable in differentiating between a full-thickness macular hole, lamellar hole, macular hole RD, and macular foveoschisis.

5. Enlargement of the subarachnoid space (SAS). Using SS-OCT, enlarged SAS was detected in 124 of 133 myopic eyes (93%). This appears as a hyporeflective triangle containing weakly hyperreflective arachnoid trabeculae, with the base toward the eye and the apex toward the optic nerve. It is postulated that enlarged SAS results in an expanded area of optic nerve exposed to cerebrospinal pressure, together with the thinning of the posterior eye wall that increases the pressure load on the peripapillary sclera, and may potentially increase susceptibility to glaucoma and visual field defects in these patients with pathological myopia [71].

6. Intrachoroidal cavitations (ICCs) appear as a hyporeflective cavity under the RPE on OCT. Occasionally, a triangular thickening near the border of the optic nerve is recognizable and has been interpreted as residual of tissue of Jacoby. ICCs have a prevalence of around 4.9–9.4% in pathological myopia. It is hypothesized that ICCs is the result of vitreal fluid dissection in eyes where there are full-thickness retinal defects over the lesion, where a direct connection between vitreous and choroid is established [72].

7. Optic disc clefts. Using SS-OCT, pit-like clefts at the outer border of the optic disc or within the adjacent scleral crescent were detected in 32 (16.2%) of 198 highly myopic eyes. These pits were situated either in the optic disc area (optic disc pits) or in the conus area (conus pits) outside the optic disc. Discontinuity of the lamina cribrosa contributed to the formation of optic disc pits, whereas conus pits appeared to develop from a scleral stretch-associated schisis or emissary openings for the short posterior ciliary arteries in the sclera. There was discontinuity of the nerve fiber layer overlying the pits, which might explain the cause of visual field defects in highly myopic individuals in these cases. The locations of the

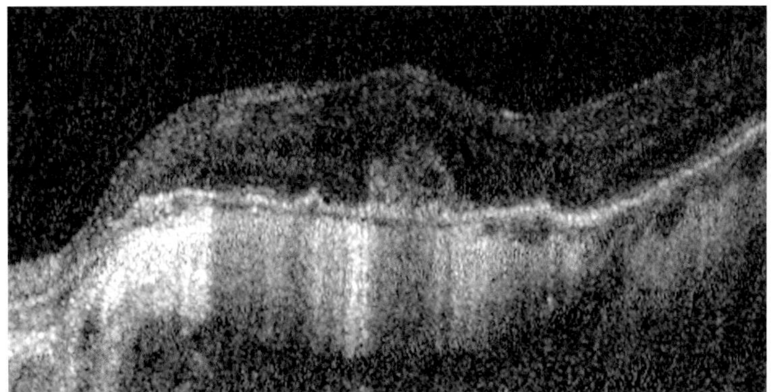

Fig. 14. Myopic choroidal neovascularization (CNV). Optical coherence tomography (OCT) scan showing subretinal hyperreflectivity corresponding to type 2 CNV lesion. Other features of myopia such as a thin choroid and optic disc excavation are also seen.

conus pits might partly explain why the papillomacular bundles tend to be damaged in highly myopic eyes [73].

Myopic CNV
Myopic CNV has a prevalence of 5–11% of individuals with high myopia [64–66, 74].

Active myopic CNV is detected on OCT by the presence of a hyperreflective lesion with indistinct, fuzzy borders in the subretinal space above the RPE (type 2 CNV) (Fig. 14). This may be associated with subretinal fluid, intraretinal fluid and exudation, and ellipsoid zone disruption [66, 75, 76]. In contrast, type 1 CNV (located in the sub-RPE space) is uncommon among eyes with myopic CNV [77]. In addition, the choroid, which is already thin among eyes with high myopia [3, 78, 79], has been shown to be thinner in eyes with myopic CNV compared to the contralateral (unaffected) eye [80].

Following treatment with anti-VEGF, the fuzzy border of the CNV lesion becomes more distinct. This is associated with thickening of the RPE, and suggests formation of a scar. In the atrophic stages, CNV fibrosis becomes flat and surrounded by an area of choriocapillary atrophy and retinal thinning [75].

In addition to diagnosis and localization of the myopic CNV lesion, OCT has been shown to be useful in monitoring the disease progress and for treatment decision-making. In the RADIANCE study [81], patients in group 2 were treated with intravitreal ranibizumab based on disease activity on OCT (defined as visual impairment attributable to intraretinal or subretinal fluid). Patients in this group gained 14.4 letters at month 12, and this was demonstrated to be noninferior to the group treated based on stabilization of visual criteria.

Conclusion

OCT provides both structural and quantitative analysis of retinal diseases and is essential for the management of patients with retinal diseases. An understanding of the anatomic changes associated with various retinal diseases can help the ophthalmologist diagnose the disease and monitor its course following treatment.

Disclosure Statement

Colin S. Tan: Research Support from National Medical Research Council Transition Award (NMRC/TA/0039/2015). Conference support from Bayer and Novartis.

Srinivas R. Sadda: Consultant for Allegan, Genentech, Roche, Novartis, Iconic, Thrombogenics, Centervue, Heidelberg, Optos, and Carl Zeiss Meditec; research Support from Allergan, Genentech, Optos, and Carl Zeiss Meditec.

References

1 Huang D, Swanson EA, Lin CP, Schuman JS, Stinson WG, Chang W, Hee MR, Flotte T, Gregory K, Puliafito CA, et al: Optical coherence tomography. Science 1991;254:1178–1181.
2 Mansouri K, Nuyen B, N Weinreb R: Improved visualization of deep ocular structures in glaucoma using high penetration optical coherence tomography. Expert Rev Med Devices 2013;10:621–628.
3 Tan CS, Ngo WK, Cheong KX: Comparison of choroidal thicknesses using swept source and spectral domain optical coherence tomography in diseased and normal eyes. Br J Ophthalmol 2015;99:354–358.
4 Tan CS, Chan JC, Cheong KX, Ngo WK, Sadda SR: Comparison of retinal thicknesses measured using swept-source and spectral-domain optical coherence tomography devices. Ophthalmic Surg Lasers Imaging Retina 2015;46:172–179.
5 Tan CS, Li KZ, Lim TH: A novel technique of adjusting segmentation boundary layers to achieve comparability of retinal thickness and volumes between spectral domain and time domain optical coherence tomography. Invest Ophthalmol Vis Sci 2012;53:5515–5519.
6 Tan CS, Li KZ, Lim TH: Calculating the predicted retinal thickness from spectral domain and time domain optical coherence tomography – comparison of different methods. Graefes Arch Clin Exp Ophthalmol 2014;252:1491–1499.
7 Flores-Moreno I, Ruiz-Medrano J, Duker JS, Ruiz-Moreno JM: The relationship between retinal and choroidal thickness and visual acuity in highly myopic eyes. Br J Ophthalmol 2013;97:1010–1013.
8 Singh N, Rohatgi J, Gupta VP, Kumar V: Measurement of peripapillary retinal nerve fiber layer thickness and macular thickness in anisometropia using spectral domain optical coherence tomography: a prospective study. Clin Ophthalmol 2017;11:429–434.
9 Tan CS, Li KZ, Tan M, Yang A, Lim LW, Zhao P, Tan M, Nah G, Tey F, Cheng CY, et al: Relationship between myopia severity and macular retinal thickness on visual performance under different lighting conditions. Ophthalmol Retina 2017;1:339–346.
10 Hwang YH, Kim YY: Macular thickness and volume of myopic eyes measured using spectral-domain optical coherence tomography. Clin Exp Optometry 2012;95:492–498.
11 Lam DS, Leung KS, Mohamed S, Chan WM, Palanivelu MS, Cheung CY, Li EY, Lai RY, Leung CK: Regional variations in the relationship between macular thickness measurements and myopia. Invest Ophthalmol Vis Sci 2007;48:376–382.
12 Tan CS, Ouyang Y, Ruiz H, Sadda SR: Diurnal variation of choroidal thickness in normal, healthy subjects measured by spectral domain optical coherence tomography. Invest Ophthalmol Vis Sci 2012;53:261–266.
13 Cicinelli MV, Rabiolo A, Sacconi R, Carnevali A, Querques L, Bandello F, Querques G: Optical coherence tomography angiography in dry age-related macular degeneration. Surv Ophthalmol 2018;63:236–244.
14 Mimoun G, Soubrane G, Coscas G: Macular drusen (in French). J Fr Ophtalmol 1990;13:511–530.
15 Arnold JJ, Sarks SH, Killingsworth MC, Sarks JP: Reticular pseudodrusen. A risk factor in age-related maculopathy. Retina 1995;15:183–191.
16 Sarks J, Arnold J, Ho IV, Sarks S, Killingsworth M: Evolution of reticular pseudodrusen. Br J Ophthalmol 2011;95:979–985.
17 Giovannini A, Amato GP, Mariotti C, Scassellati-Sforzolini B: OCT imaging of choroidal neovascularisation and its role in the determination of patients' eligibility for surgery. Br J Ophthalmol 1999;83:438–442.
18 Yannuzzi LA, Sorenson J, Spaide RF, Lipson B: Idiopathic polypoidal choroidal vasculopathy (IPCV). 1990. Retina 2012;32(suppl 1):1–8.
19 Imamura Y, Engelbert M, Iida T, Freund KB, Yannuzzi LA: Polypoidal choroidal vasculopathy: a review. Surv Ophthalmol 2010;55:501–515.
20 Lim TH, Laude A, Tan CS: Polypoidal choroidal vasculopathy: an angiographic discussion. Eye (Lond) 2010;24:483–490.
21 Tan CS, Ngo WK, Chen JP, Tan NW, Lim TH: EVEREST study report 2: imaging and grading protocol, and baseline characteristics of a randomised controlled trial of polypoidal choroidal vasculopathy. Br J Ophthalmol 2015;99:624–628.
22 Koh A, Lai TYY, Takahashi K, Wong TY, Chen LJ, Ruamviboonsuk P, Tan CS, Feller C, Margaron P, Lim TH, et al: Efficacy and safety of ranibizumab with or without verteporfin photodynamic therapy for polypoidal choroidal vasculopathy: a randomized clinical trial. JAMA Ophthalmol 2017;135:1206–1213.
23 Koh A, Lee WK, Chen LJ, Chen SJ, Hashad Y, Kim H, Lai TY, Pilz S, Ruamviboonsuk P, Tokaji E, et al: EVEREST study: efficacy and safety of verteporfin photodynamic therapy in combination with ranibizumab or alone versus ranibizumab monotherapy in patients with symptomatic macular polypoidal choroidal vasculopathy. Retina 2012;32:1453–1464.
24 Tan CS, Ngo WK, Lim LW, Lim TH: A novel classification of the vascular patterns of polypoidal choroidal vasculopathy and its relation to clinical outcomes. Br J Ophthalmol 2014;98:1528–1533.
25 Tan CS, Ngo WK, Lim LW, Tan NW, Lim TH; EVEREST Study Group: EVEREST study report 3: diagnostic challenges of polypoidal choroidal vasculopathy. Lessons learnt from screening failures in the EVEREST study. Graefes Arch Clin Exp Ophthalmol 2016;254:1923–1930.
26 Chang YS, Kim JH, Kim JW, Lee TG, Kim CG: Optical coherence tomography-based diagnosis of polypoidal choroidal vasculopathy in Korean patients. Korean J Ophthalmol 2016;30:198–205.
27 De Salvo G, Vaz-Pereira S, Keane PA, Tufail A, Liew G: Sensitivity and specificity of spectral-domain optical coherence tomography in detecting idiopathic polypoidal choroidal vasculopathy. Am J Ophthalmol 2014;158:1228–1238.e1221.
28 Sa HS, Cho HY, Kang SW: Optical coherence tomography of idiopathic polypoidal choroidal vasculopathy. Korean J Ophthalmol 2005;19:275–280.

29 Iijima H, Iida T, Imai M, Gohdo T, Tsukahara S: Optical coherence tomography of orange-red subretinal lesions in eyes with idiopathic polypoidal choroidal vasculopathy. Am J Ophthalmol 2000; 129:21–26.

30 Kawamura A, Yuzawa M, Mori R, Haruyama M, Tanaka K: Indocyanine green angiographic and optical coherence tomographic findings support classification of polypoidal choroidal vasculopathy into two types. Acta Ophthalmol 2013;91:e474–e481.

31 Ozawa S, Ishikawa K, Ito Y, Nishihara H, Yamakoshi T, Hatta Y, Terasaki H: Differences in macular morphology between polypoidal choroidal vasculopathy and exudative age-related macular degeneration detected by optical coherence tomography. Retina 2009;29:793–802.

32 Sato T, Kishi S, Watanabe G, Matsumoto H, Mukai R: Tomographic features of branching vascular networks in polypoidal choroidal vasculopathy. Retina 2007; 27:589–594.

33 Liu R, Li J, Li Z, Yu S, Yang Y, Yan H, Zeng J, Tang S, Ding X: Distinguishing polypoidal choroidal vasculopathy from typical neovascular age-related macular degeneration based on spectral domain optical coherence tomography. Retina 2016;36:778–786.

34 Koizumi H, Yamagishi T, Yamazaki T, Kawasaki R, Kinoshita S: Subfoveal choroidal thickness in typical age-related macular degeneration and polypoidal choroidal vasculopathy. Graefes Arch Clin Exp Ophthalmol 2011;249:1123–1128.

35 Alshahrani ST, Al Shamsi HN, Kahtani ES, Ghazi NG: Spectral-domain optical coherence tomography findings in polypoidal choroidal vasculopathy suggest a type 1 neovascular growth pattern. Clin Ophthalmol 2014;8:1689–1695.

36 Cho M, Athanikar A, Paccione J, Wald KJ: Optical coherence tomography features of acute central serous chorioretinopathy versus neovascular age-related macular degeneration. Br J Ophthalmol 2010;94:597–599.

37 Fujimoto H, Gomi F, Wakabayashi T, Sawa M, Tsujikawa M, Tano Y: Morphologic changes in acute central serous chorioretinopathy evaluated by Fourier-domain optical coherence tomography. Ophthalmology 2008;115:1494–1500, 1500.e1491–1492.

38 Imamura Y, Fujiwara T, Margolis R, Spaide RF: Enhanced depth imaging optical coherence tomography of the choroid in central serous chorioretinopathy. Retina 2009;29:1469–1473.

39 Ojima Y, Hangai M, Sasahara M, Gotoh N, Inoue R, Yasuno Y, Makita S, Yatagai T, Tsujikawa A, Yoshimura N: Three-dimensional imaging of the foveal photoreceptor layer in central serous chorioretinopathy using high-speed optical coherence tomography. Ophthalmology 2007;114:2197–2207.

40 Kim BY, Smith SD, Kaiser PK: Optical coherence tomographic patterns of diabetic macular edema. Am J Ophthalmol 2006;142:405–412.

41 Kim NR, Kim YJ, Chin HS, Moon YS: Optical coherence tomographic patterns in diabetic macular oedema: prediction of visual outcome after focal laser photocoagulation. Br J Ophthalmol 2009;93: 901–905.

42 Otani T, Kishi S, Maruyama Y: Patterns of diabetic macular edema with optical coherence tomography. Am J Ophthalmol 1999;127:688–693.

43 Browning DJ, Glassman AR, Aiello LP, Beck RW, Brown DM, Fong DS, Bressler NM, Danis RP, Kinyoun JL, Nguyen QD, et al: Relationship between optical coherence tomography-measured central retinal thickness and visual acuity in diabetic macular edema. Ophthalmology 2007;114:525–536.

44 Ozdek SC, Erdinc MA, Gurelik G, Aydin B, Bahceci U, Hasanreisoglu B: Optical coherence tomographic assessment of diabetic macular edema: comparison with fluorescein angiographic and clinical findings. Ophthalmologica 2005;219: 86–92.

45 Yeung L, Lima VC, Garcia P, Landa G, Rosen RB: Correlation between spectral domain optical coherence tomography findings and fluorescein angiography patterns in diabetic macular edema. Ophthalmology 2009;116:1158–1167.

46 Lang GE: Optical coherence tomography findings in diabetic retinopathy. Dev Ophthalmol 2007;39:31–47.

47 Ghazi NG, Ciralsky JB, Shah SM, Campochiaro PA, Haller JA: Optical coherence tomography findings in persistent diabetic macular edema: the vitreomacular interface. Am J Ophthalmol 2007; 144:747–754.

48 Gallemore RP, Jumper JM, McCuen BW 2nd, Jaffe GJ, Postel EA, Toth CA: Diagnosis of vitreoretinal adhesions in macular disease with optical coherence tomography. Retina 2000;20:115–120.

49 Massin P, Duguid G, Erginay A, Haouchine B, Gaudric A: Optical coherence tomography for evaluating diabetic macular edema before and after vitrectomy. Am J Ophthalmol 2003;135:169–177.

50 Wilkins JR, Puliafito CA, Hee MR, Duker JS, Reichel E, Coker JG, Schuman JS, Swanson EA, Fujimoto JG: Characterization of epiretinal membranes using optical coherence tomography. Ophthalmology 1996;103:2142–2151.

51 Kang SW, Park CY, Ham DI: The correlation between fluorescein angiographic and optical coherence tomographic features in clinically significant diabetic macular edema. Am J Ophthalmol 2004; 137:313–322.

52 Soliman W, Sander B, Jorgensen TM: Enhanced optical coherence patterns of diabetic macular oedema and their correlation with the pathophysiology. Acta Ophthalmol Scand 2007;85:613–617.

53 Muraoka Y, Uji A, Tsujikawa A, Murakami T, Ooto S, Suzuma K, Takahashi A, Iida Y, Miwa Y, Hata M, et al: Association between retinal hemorrhagic pattern and macular perfusion status in eyes with acute branch retinal vein occlusion. Sci Rep 2016;6:28554.

54 Ko J, Kwon OW, Byeon SH: Optical coherence tomography predicts visual outcome in acute central retinal vein occlusion. Retina 2014;34:1132–1141.

55 Rahimy E, Sarraf D, Dollin ML, Pitcher JD, Ho AC: Paracentral acute middle maculopathy in nonischemic central retinal vein occlusion. Am J Ophthalmol 2014;158:372–380.e371.

56 Schroder K, Ackermann P, Brachert M, Bairov S, Geerling G, Guthoff R: Does OCT morphology provide indications for prognosis of visual acuity after venous occlusion? SD-OCT analysis in retinal vein occlusion before and after resolution of initial macular edema (in German). Ophthalmologe 2016;113: 500–506.

57 Ozdemir H, Karacorlu M, Karacorlu SA, Senturk F: Localized foveal detachment in a patient with central retinal artery occlusion with cilioretinal sparing. Eur J Ophthalmol 2012;22:492–494.

58 Ozdemir H, Karacorlu S, Karacorlu M: Optical coherence tomography findings in central retinal artery occlusion. Retina 2006;26:110–112.

59 Chen SN, Hwang JF, Chen YT: Macular thickness measurements in central retinal artery occlusion by optical coherence tomography. Retina 2011;31:730–737.

60 Dolar-Szczasny J, Swiech-Zubilewicz A, Oleszczuk A, Mackiewicz J: Optical coherence tomography (OCT) examination in patients with central retinal artery occlusion (in Polish). Klin Oczna 2012;114:26–28.

61 Shinoda K, Yamada K, Matsumoto CS, Kimoto K, Nakatsuka K: Changes in retinal thickness are correlated with alterations of electroretinogram in eyes with central retinal artery occlusion. Graefes Arch Clin Exp Ophthalmol 2008;246:949–954.

62 Yu S, Pang CE, Gong Y, Freund KB, Yannuzzi LA, Rahimy E, Lujan BJ, Tabandeh H, Cooney MJ, Sarraf D: The spectrum of superficial and deep capillary ischemia in retinal artery occlusion. Am J Ophthalmol 2015;159:53–63.e51–e52.

63 Lin LL, Shih YF, Hsiao CK, Chen CJ: Prevalence of myopia in Taiwanese schoolchildren: 1983 to 2000. Ann Acad Med Singapore 2004;33:27–33.

64 Wong TY, Ferreira A, Hughes R, Carter G, Mitchell P: Epidemiology and disease burden of pathologic myopia and myopic choroidal neovascularization: an evidence-based systematic review. Am J Ophthalmol 2014;157:9–25.e12.

65 Wong TY, Foster PJ, Hee J, Ng TP, Tielsch JM, Chew SJ, Johnson GJ, Seah SK: Prevalence and risk factors for refractive errors in adult Chinese in Singapore. Investigative Ophthalmol Vis Sci 2000; 41:2486–2494.

66 Ohno-Matsui K, Lai TY, Lai CC, Cheung CM: Updates of pathologic myopia. Prog Retin Eye Res 2016;52:156–187.

67 Gaucher D, Erginay A, Lecleire-Collet A, Haouchine B, Puech M, Cohen SY, Massin P, Gaudric A: Dome-shaped macula in eyes with myopic posterior staphyloma. Am J Ophthalmol 2008;145:909–914.

68 Imamura Y, Iida T, Maruko I, Zweifel SA, Spaide RF: Enhanced depth imaging optical coherence tomography of the sclera in dome-shaped macula. Am J Ophthalmol 2011;151:297–302.

69 Coco RM, Sanabria MR, Alegria J: Pathology associated with optical coherence tomography macular bending due to either dome-shaped macula or inferior staphyloma in myopic patients. Ophthalmologica 2012;228:7–12.

70 Sun CB, Liu Z, Xue AQ, Yao K: Natural evolution from macular retinoschisis to full-thickness macular hole in highly myopic eyes. Eye (Lond) 2010;24:1787–1791.

71 Ohno-Matsui K, Akiba M, Moriyama M, Ishibashi T, Tokoro T, Spaide RF: Imaging retrobulbar subarachnoid space around optic nerve by swept-source optical coherence tomography in eyes with pathologic myopia. Invest Ophthalmol Vis Sci 2011;52:9644–9650.

72 Spaide RF, Akiba M, Ohno-Matsui K: Evaluation of peripapillary intrachoroidal cavitation with swept source and enhanced depth imaging optical coherence tomography. Retina 2012;32:1037–1044.

73 Ohno-Matsui K, Akiba M, Moriyama M, Shimada N, Ishibashi T, Tokoro T, Spaide RF: Acquired optic nerve and peripapillary pits in pathologic myopia. Ophthalmology 2012;119:1685–1692.

74 Tan CS, Chew MC, Lim TH: Comparison of foveal-sparing with foveal-involving photodynamic therapy for myopic choroidal neovascularization. Eye (Lond) 2014;28:17–22.

75 Introini U, Casalino G, Querques G, Gimeno AT, Scotti F, Bandello F: Spectral-domain OCT in anti-VEGF treatment of myopic choroidal neovascularization. Eye (Lond) 2012;26:976–982.

76 Jonas JB, Jonas SB, Jonas RA, Holbach L, Dai Y, Sun X, Panda-Jonas S: Parapapillary atrophy: histological gamma zone and delta zone. PLoS One 2012; 7:e47237.

77 Silva R: Myopic maculopathy: a review. Ophthalmologica 2012;228:197–213.

78 Tan CS, Cheong KX: Macular choroidal thicknesses in healthy adults – relationship with ocular and demographic factors. Invest Ophthalmol Vis Sci 2014;55: 6452–6458.

79 Tan CS, Cheong KX, Lim LW, Li KZ: Topographic variation of choroidal and retinal thicknesses at the macula in healthy adults. Br J Ophthalmol 2014;98: 339–344.

80 Ikuno Y, Jo Y, Hamasaki T, Tano Y: Ocular risk factors for choroidal neovascularization in pathologic myopia. Invest Ophthalmol Vis Sci 2010;51:3721–3725.

81 Wolf S, Balciuniene VJ, Laganovska G, Menchini U, Ohno-Matsui K, Sharma T, Wong TY, Silva R, Pilz S, Gekkieva M: RADIANCE: a randomized controlled study of ranibizumab in patients with choroidal neovascularization secondary to pathologic myopia. Ophthalmology 2014;121:682–692.e682.

Colin S. Tan
National Healthcare Group Eye Institute
Tan Tock Seng Hospital
11 Jalan Tan Tock Seng
Singapore 308433 (Singapore)
E-Mail colintan_eye@yahoo.com.sg

Cunha-Vaz J, Koh A (eds): Imaging Techniques.
ESASO Course Series. Basel, Karger, 2018, vol 10, pp 37–51 (DOI: 10.1159/000487411)

Optical Coherence Tomography: Choroidal Imaging

Anna C.S. Tan[a–d] · K. Bailey Freund[a, b, e] · Lawrence A. Yannuzzi[a, b]

[a]Vitreous, Retina Macula, Consultants of New York, and [b]LuEsther T Mertz Retinal Research Center, Manhattan, Eye, Ear and Throat Hospital, New York, NY, USA; [c]Singapore National Eye Center/Singapore Eye Research Institute, and [d]Duke-NUS Medical School, Singapore, Singapore; [e]Department of Ophthalmology, New York University School of Medicine, New York, NY, USA

Abstract

The choroid has an important role in supporting the retinal pigment epithelium and photoreceptor layers and is responsible for maintaining normal retinal function. Pathological changes in the choroid that can be detected by optical coherence tomography (OCT) are observed in diseases such as age-related macular degeneration, pachychoroid disease (e.g., central serous chorioretinopathy, pachychoroid neovasculopathy, and polypoidal choroidal vasculopathy), myopic degeneration, inflammatory disease, inherited retinal and choroidal dystrophies, as well as in choroidal tumors. A quick, noninvasive form of imaging, OCT shows good reproducibility over various platforms and allows consecutive imaging of eyes during the course of follow-up to monitor disease progression and detect recurrence. Advances in OCT imaging combined with the advent of antiangiogenic therapies have revolutionized the treatment of many common retinal diseases. Novel OCT imaging techniques such as enhanced-depth imaging OCT and new technology including swept-source OCT enable enhanced choroidal imaging. These advances can be used to correlate structure with histology, thereby enhancing our understanding of disease pathogenesis. Other developments such as three-dimensional OCT imaging and more reliable tissue segmentation algorithms can produce en face OCT images with automated analysis and quantification of various retinal and choroidal parameters which are useful for both clinical and research applications.

Optical coherence tomography (OCT) imaging, an easy to perform noninvasive test, has allowed choroidal structures and pathology to be studied in more detail than ever before. Previous imaging of the choroid revolved around techniques such as indocyanine green angiography (ICGA) [1, 2], laser Doppler flowmetry and ultrasound [3]. These techniques allow imaging of the cho-

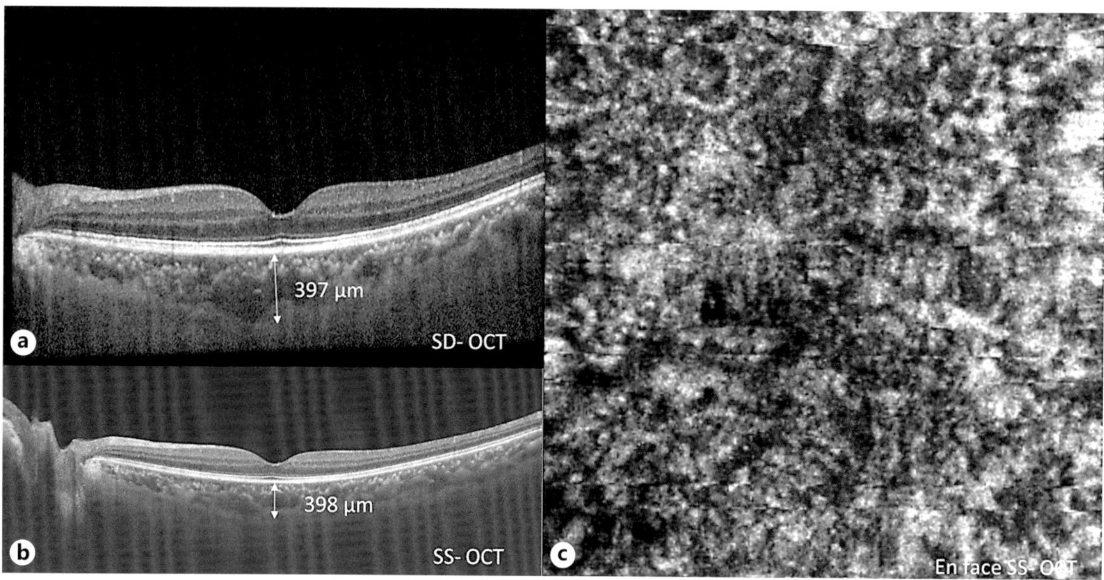

Fig. 1. Comparison of spectral-domain optical coherence tomography (OCT; **a**) with swept-source (SS)-OCT (**b**) in the same eye and a corresponding en face SS-OCT (**c**). Subfoveal choroidal thickness measurements are shown by the white double-headed arrows.

roidal vasculature and choroidal blood flow, while OCT has the unique advantage of allowing depth-resolved, three-dimensional imaging of the retina, retinal pigment epithelium (RPE), and choroid [3].

The evolution from time-domain OCT, to spectral-domain (SD)-OCT and then to swept-source (SS)-OCT has shown rapid improvements in the scanning rates, resolution and width and the depth of field (Fig. 1) [4]. Additional advances such as denser raster scans, more varied scan patterns, enhanced image quality, better reproducibility, volumetric datasets and the ability to view both cross-sectional and en face OCT images has significantly improved our understanding of choroidal diseases [4]. In particular, enhanced-depth imaging (EDI)-OCT has enabled reproducible images of the choroid that can be quantified and monitored during disease progression [5, 6]. The role of the choroid is to provide the vascular supply, oxygen, growth factors, and other nutrients to the outer retina including the photoreceptors.

Pathological changes detected in the choroid on OCT have been seen in conditions such as age-related macular degeneration (AMD) [7, 8], pachychoroid diseases such as polypoidal choroidal vasculopathy (PCV) [9] or central serous chorioretinopathy [9], pathological myopia [10], inflammatory diseases, and choroidal tumors [11]. High-resolution OCT images have enabled imaging-histology correlations to identify specific pathological changes occurring in the choroid at the microscopic level [12, 13].

OCT of the Choroid in Normal Eyes

Choroidal thickness on OCT has been defined by the perpendicular distance from the outer edge of the hyperreflective RPE/Bruch's complex to the inner sclera or choroid-sclera junction (Fig. 1). Good reproducibility has been found between measurements obtained using various SD-OCT systems (e.g., Spectralis, Cirrus, and RTvue) in

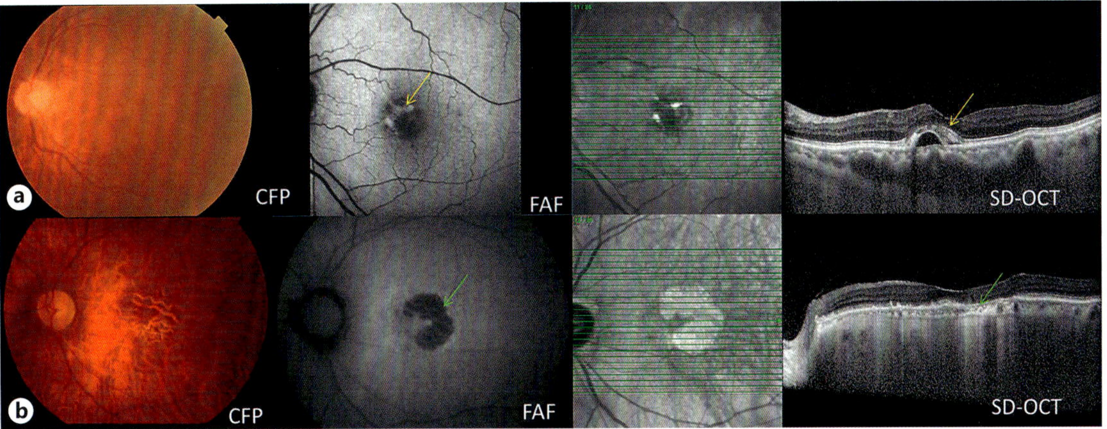

Fig. 2. An eye with intermediate age-related macular degeneration (**a**), with a pigment epithelial detachment. A hyperreflective overlying acquired vitelliform lesion (yellow arrows) corresponds to the area of hyperautofluorescence. An eye with geographic atrophy shows loss of the retinal pigment epithelium and outer retinal bands producing choroidal hypertransmission (**b**, green arrows). CFP, color fundus photograph; FAF, fundus autofluorescence; SD-OCT, spectral-domain OCT.

eyes of young healthy volunteers. In normal eyes, the mean subfoveal choroidal thickness reported in studies ranged from 272 to 279 μm on SD-OCT [14] and from 279 to 285 μm on SS-OCT [14], with good interdevice correlation between the SD-OCT and SS-OCT systems [14, 15]. Topographic measurements of the choroidal thickness of the macula showed that the choroid was thickest at the subfoveal area and thinnest at the region nasal to the fovea [16]. Mean choroidal thickness decreases with increasing axial length and with advancing age [17].

OCT and AMD

OCT is an integral part of multimodal imaging and its use in combination with color fundus photos (CFP), fundus autofluorescence (FAF), fluorescein angiography (FA), and ICGA is the standard of care to evaluate AMD [18]. AMD, characterized by aging changes in the retina, the presence of drusen and often a reduced choroidal thickness, can be broadly classified into early, intermediate, and late or advanced AMD [19]. Advanced AMD includes either "dry" or non-neovascular AMD characterized by geographic atrophy (GA) of the macula, while "wet" or neovascular AMD is characterized by the development of neovascularization (NV) beneath or within the retina resulting in exudation, hemorrhage, pigment epithelial detachments (PEDs) and subsequent fibrosis and scarring [19].

OCT and Non-Neovascular AMD

In non-neovascular AMD, drusen and larger drusenoid PEDs appear on cross-sectional OCT imaging as discrete lobular detachments of the RPE with underlying homogenous, hyperreflective contents affecting the central macula. Intraretinal or subretinal fluid overlying drusenoid PEDs is usually not observed. Pigmentary changes and vitelliform detachments overlying the PED can appear as intraretinal and subretinal hyperreflective material on OCT respectively (Fig. 2a). Consistent with previous studies, the choroid is generally thin in these patients [20]; however, this may vary according to various drusen subtypes (Fig. 2b). Reticular pseudodrusen, in particular, are associated with a thin choroid [21], while in eyes with cuticular drusen and vitelliform detachment, a thicker choroid (Fig. 2a) is observed when compared to eyes with cuticular drusen alone [22]. One study comparing choroidal thickness of healthy subjects with that of patients with bilateral intermediate AMD and that of patients with intermediate AMD in one eye and neovascular AMD in the fellow eye, found that that patients with unilateral AMD had the thinnest choroids [23].

During the intermediate progression of non-neovascular AMD, visible disruption of the hyperreflective RPE band was seen with OCT preceding the spontaneous collapse of drusenoid PEDs that often resulted in GA (Fig. 2b) [24]. In eyes with GA, widespread choroidal thinning was observed independent of the area of retinal pigment atrophy, and this correlated with both subfoveal large choroidal vessel layer thickness and medium choroidal vessel layer/choriocapillaris layer thickness [25]. Reduced choroidal thickness has been associated with increased hyperreflectivity of GA on near-infrared imaging [26]. Subfoveal choroidal thickness measured by OCT is closely related to visual outcomes, including severity of non-neovascular AMD and rate of GA progression [27]. FAF has emerged as an important outcome measure for many GA interventional trials, and en face OCT analyzed at the outer retinal layer but not at the choroidal layer showed good correlation with the areas of hypoautofluorescence on FAF (Fig. 2b, second column) [28].

OCT and Neovascular AMD
Multimodal imaging has identified three types of NV in AMD based on their anatomical location within the retinal and subretinal layers [29]: type 1 NV is NV located between the RPE and Bruch's membrane and is associated with vascularized PEDs, type 2 NV is NV located in the subretinal space above the RPE and type 3 NV, also known as retinal angiomatous proliferation, is intraretinal NV (Fig. 3).

On OCT imaging, type 1 NV or vascularized PEDs have less defined margins, uneven surfaces and an irregular shape (Fig. 3a). The appearance of the contents of the vascularized PED vary on OCT, and a previous study using EDI-OCT imaging showed that in about half of these vascularized PEDs, the entire PED cavity was filled with highly hyperreflective material, while the other half had heterogeneous collections of serous fluid and hyperreflective material [6]. The hyperreflective material that was located on the basal surface of the RPE was likely fibrovascular proliferation that sometimes appears elevated above Bruch's membrane on OCT [6]. In some cases, an "onion sign," is observed within vascularized PEDs, which has been histologically correlated with cholesterol deposition within the lesion (Fig. 3) [30]. The choroid in patients with vascularized PEDs is usually thin compared to healthy eyes [20]; however, previous studies showed that increased subfoveal choroidal thickness may be associated with better visual outcomes in eyes with type 1 NV [31] (Fig. 3a).

Type 2 NV on OCT imaging appears as subretinal hyperreflective material seen in the subretinal space above the RPE [32]. The appearance of type 2 NV on both two- and three-dimensional OCT imaging was described as having well-defined steep margins with a crater-like configuration showing good correlation with FA patterns (Fig. 3b) [33]. The OCT appearance of type 3 NV has been described as a central hyperreflective funnel-like lesions above the PED that appears to have originated in the deep vascular complex [29, 34] (Fig. 3c). This intraretinal hyperreflective structure bordered by intraretinal cystic changes forms a "mask"-like appearance on OCT [34, 35] (Fig. 3c). Progression of type 3 NV may be associated with a focal RPE defect at the apex of an underlying drusenoid PED, which then develops a serous component. The choroid of eyes developing type 3 NV is often thinner than that seen in eyes with other lesion compositions, and focal areas of atrophy may be seen on both OCT and FAF imaging [36] (Fig. 3b).

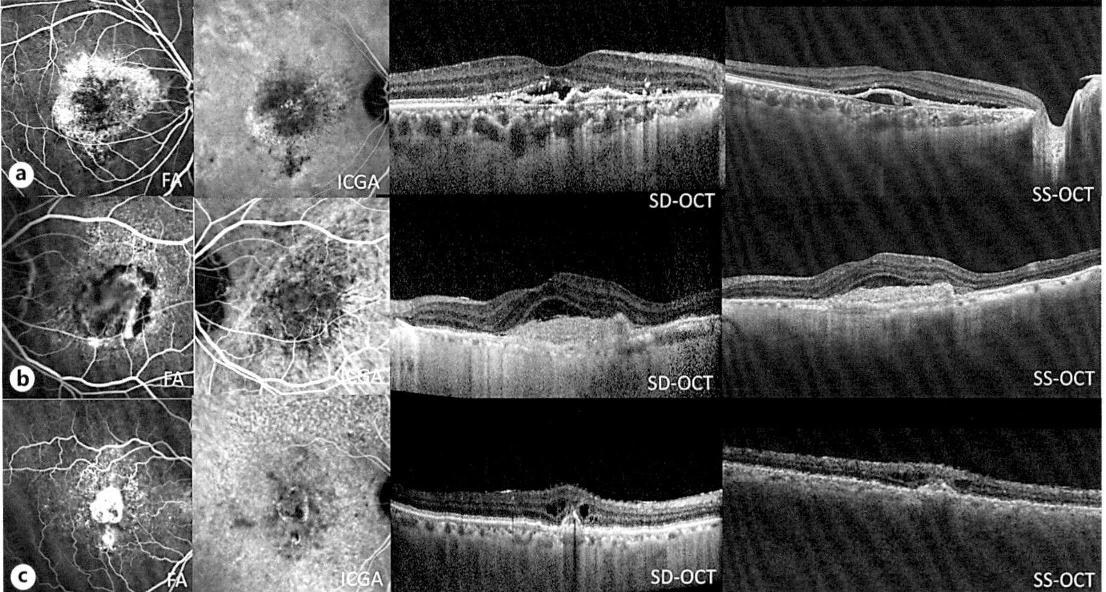

Fig. 3. Multimodal imaging of type 1 neovascularization (NV) (**a**), type 2 NV (**b**) and type 3 NV (**c**). Type 1 NV is characterized by late leakage on fluorescein angiography (FA), a plaque on indocyanine green angiography (ICGA) and a vascularized pigment epithelial detachment with hyperreflective contents on optical coherence tomography (OCT). Type 2 NV is characterized by early leakage on FA, an area of blocked cyanescence on ICGA and subretinal hyperreflective material on OCT. Type 3 NV is characterized by focal leakage on FA seen below the area of atrophy, ICGA showing a right-angled vessel and OCT showing intraretinal hyperreflective linear structure with surrounding intraretinal fluid. SD-OCT, spectral-domain OCT; SS-OCT, swept-source OCT.

The emergence of OCT technology paired with the introduction of intravitreal antiangiogenic therapy for the treatment of neovascular AMD and other vascular endothelial growth factor (VEGF)-mediated diseases, allowed OCT outcome measures to be developed to monitor the progression of disease and to detect early recurrences even before the visual acuity was affected [4, 37]. For the monitoring of disease progression, changes in the macular retinal thickness maps and central subfoveal thickness of the retina were observed in response to treatment. In addition, choroidal thickness measured on OCT has also been shown to decrease in response to the intravitreal anti-VEGF treatment for AMD [8, 38]. One study reported that afibercept showed a greater reduction of choroidal thickness than ranibizumab in eyes treated with three, monthly intravitreal injections.

OCT and Pachychoroid Diseases

Pachychoroid is a choroidal phenotype showing dilated outer choroidal (Haller's layer) veins termed "pachyvessels," inner choroidal attenuation overlying pachyvessels, hyperpermeability on ICGA, and a diffuse or focal increase in choroidal thickness. The choroidal findings of pachychoroid can be imaged with EDI-OCT, SS OCT, and with ICGA (Fig. 4) [39, 40]. Diseases such as CSC, pachychoroid neovasculopathy, and PCV have been associated with pachychoroid. Using OCT to analyze choroidal thickness and the internal structure in these entities may be useful to study the pathogenesis of these diseases and monitor disease progression (Fig. 4) [20, 39–41].

Polyps in PCV identified on ICGA can be visualized on OCT in several ways: underneath

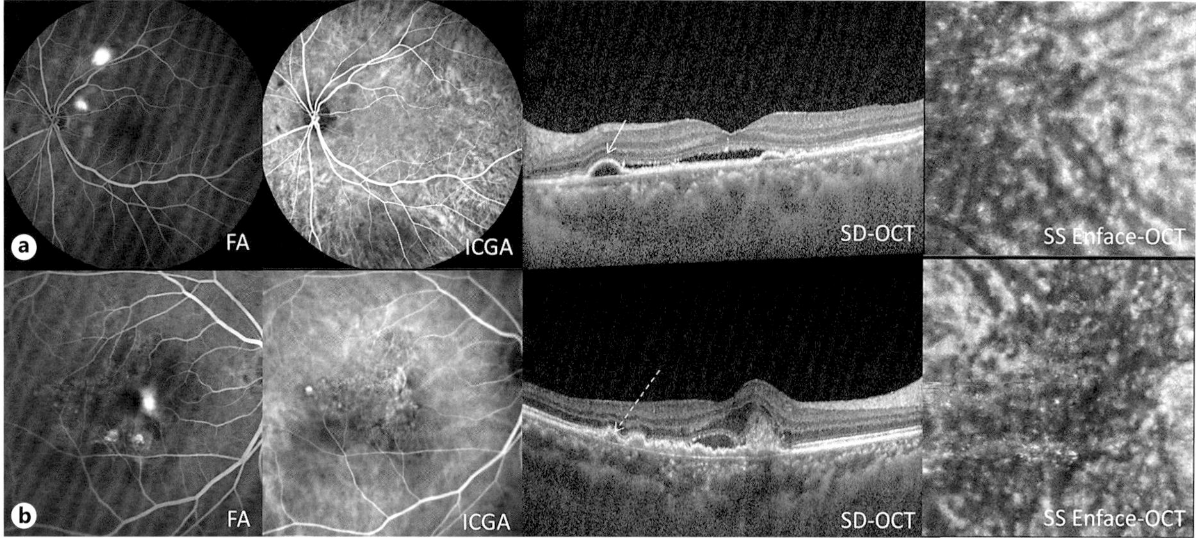

Fig. 4. Examples of eyes with pachychoroid disease; left eye with central serous chorioretinopathy (**a**), shows ink blot leakage on fluorescein angiography (FA), dilated choroidal veins (pachyvessels) and hyperpermeability on indocyanine green angiography (ICGA). There is an area of exudative subretinal fluid with an underlying serous pigment epithelial detachment (PED; non-dashed arrow). En face OCT of the choroidal vasculature shows the presence of pachyvessels. Right eye with polypoidal choroidal vasculopathy and a branching vascular network (BVN) (**b**) shows leakage on FA. The polyp is seen as an area of focal hypercyanescence on ICGA temporal to the plaque appearance of the BVN. The optical coherence tomography (OCT) of the polyp shows a peaked PED (dashed arrow) with a BVN seen as a shallow irregular PED. SD-OCT, spectral-domain OCT; SS-OCT, swept-source OCT.

the surface of a large serous PED as a series of round structures ("pearls on string appearance"), a smaller peaked PED (at the area of a notch) adjacent to a larger serous PED, or as sharp peak-like elevations within a PED with underlying moderate reflectivity (Fig. 4b) [41]. In some cases, multilayered PEDs can be observed with the elevated region of NV leaving a hyporeflective cleft over the Bruch's membrane resulting in what was described as the "triple layer sign" [30]. A normal to thick choroid with the presence of large, hyperpermeable choroidal vessels (pachyvessels) is typically present in these patients (Fig. 4b) [40, 41]. A previous study that supported these findings has shown that the subfoveal choroid in eyes with PCV is thicker (319.92 ± 68.66 μm) when compared to patients with typical AMD and no polyps (186.62 ± 64.02 μm) and normal controls (241.97 ± 66.37 μm) [41] but thinner when compared to eyes with CSC (367.81 ± 105.56 μm).

In both the active and chronic stages of CSC, a neurosensory detachment can be seen on OCT imaging (Fig. 4a). Chronic CSC can be associated with intraretinal cystic changes and may occur when there is disruption of the external limiting membrane seen on OCT. Serous PEDs associated with CSC typically show a well-circumscribed convex, dome-shaped, anterior protrusion of the RPE with a smooth surface, steep edges, and a homogenous underlying hyporeflective space on OCT (Fig. 4a). Hyperreflective material anterior to the RPE may be associated with more turbid exudation or fibrin. A thick choroid with large choroidal vessels (pachychoroid) is virtually always observed in eyes with CSC and serous PEDs (Fig. 4a) [20, 39, 41].

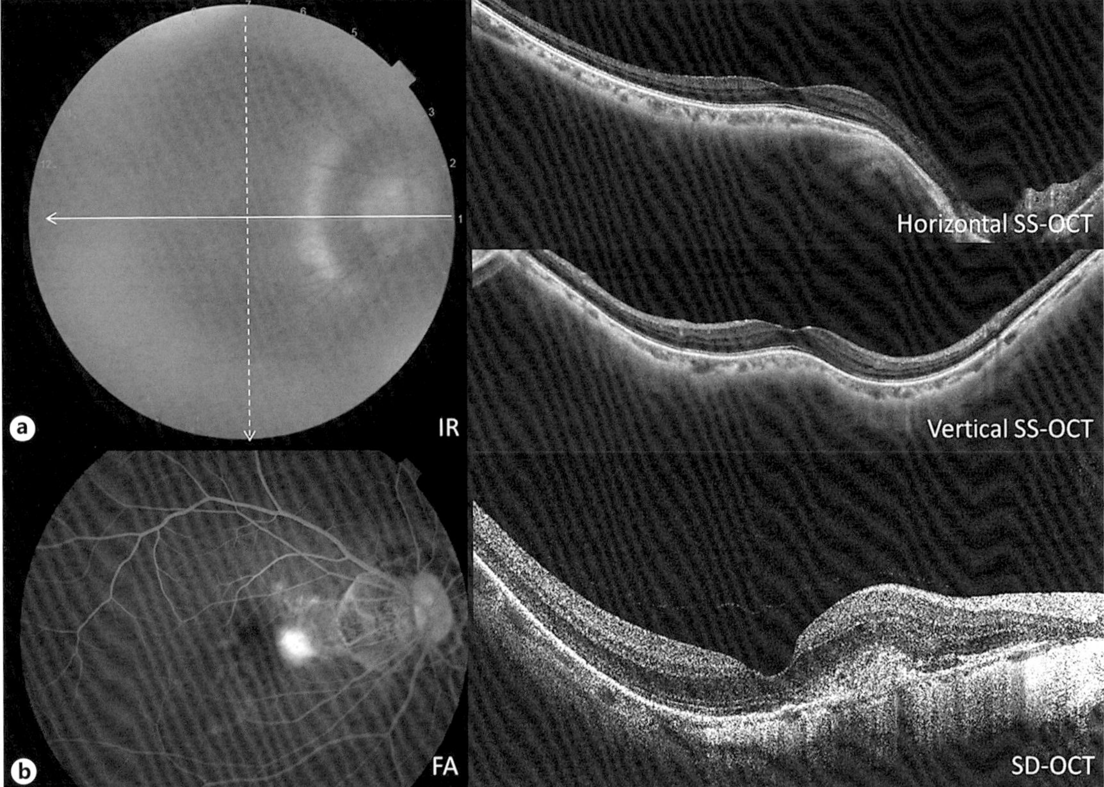

Fig. 5. Infrared (IR) image shows a myopic fundus with a tilted disc and peripapillary atrophy (**a**). Horizontal OCT shows a staphyloma, and the vertical OCT shows the presence of dome-shaped macula. Fluorescein angiography (FA) (**b**) shows myopic choroidal neovascularization with leakage and corresponding subretinal hyperreflective material seen on optical coherence tomography (OCT). SS-OCT, swept-source OCT; SD-OCT, spectral-domain OCT.

OCT and Myopia

OCT imaging in myopic eyes may be challenging due to the long axial length and steep curvature of the eye (Fig. 5). Ultrawide field OCT, in a radial pattern has been shown to be useful for imaging the entire posterior inner curvature including the staphyloma (Fig. 5) [42]. Previous studies have shown a significant correlation between increasing age and refractive error and a thinner choroid measured on OCT [43]. The development and progression of pathological myopia has been hypothesized to occur due to scleral elongation caused by growth factors secreted by the choroid, and OCT imaging has the advantage of allowing detailed in vivo choroidal details to be studied during ocular development to understand the anatomical changes that may affect emmetropization [44]. Highly myopic eyes have been associated with a thin choroid (leptochoroid) on OCT, in addition to a highly altered choroidal vasculature, especially in the presence of staphyloma [45]. SS-OCT, in conjunction with ICGA, has the potential to image other vascular structures such as posterior vortex vein ampullae, both the long and short posterior ciliary arteries and some retrobulbar vasculature (Fig. 5) [46].

Previous studies have correlated subfoveal choroidal thickness in highly myopic eyes with visual function [47]. Clinically, OCT is useful in assessing highly myopic eyes for the progression of atrophy and the development of myopic choroidal NV (mCNV) (Fig. 5b). mCNV can be characterized on OCT by the presence of subretinal hyperreflective material in association with subretinal or intraretinal fluid (Fig. 5b) [48]. Some studies show that some mCNV may show just subtle exudative changes on OCT, so FA may be more sensitive in detecting active mCNV in these eyes [49]. However, OCT can be helpful in excluding other entities in the differential diagnosis of mCNV such as macula hemorrhages, small focal areas of chorioretinal atrophy or scarring, and inflammatory conditions such as idiopathic multifocal choroiditis (MFC)/punctate inner choroidopathy (PIC) [50, 51]. OCT is useful as an outcome measure when monitoring response to intravitreal anti-VEGF therapy [52]. Characteristics on OCT of an inactive mCNV are a compact lesion, with reduced internal reflectivity compared to the surface and sharp boundaries [48]. Another important application of OCT in highly myopic eyes is the identification of intrachoroidal cavitations (ICC) located inferiorly to the optic disc. Progressive enlargement of ICC and overlying retinal thinning can cause communication of the ICC with the subretinal space resulting in a localized macular detachment [53, 54].

OCT imaging has the capability to image the sclera, which appears as a hyperreflective layer beneath the choroid. A comparative study between EDI-OCT and SS-OCT showed that in highly myopic eyes, SS-OCT was more sensitive at detecting the posterior scleral border (Fig. 5a). In addition to central retinal and choroidal thickness, other factors shown to affect the visibility of the scleral layer on OCT include age, axial length, and presence of a staphyloma [46]. Dome-shaped macula (DSM), described as an inward bulge of the macula within the concave area of the staphyloma, is an entity most readily identified using OCT (Fig. 5a). One study showed that DSM visualized by EDI-OCT was caused by localized variation in scleral thickness in the macula region. EDI-OCT was used to further classify DSM into various subtypes [55, 56]. Another study reported that eyes with staphyloma/DSM/tilted disc syndrome associated with serous retinal detachment (SRD) had a thicker subfoveal choroidal thickness, larger variations in choroidal thickness, and focal abrupt changes in choroidal thickness when compared to similar eyes without SRD [42].

OCT and Inflammatory Diseases

Choroidal OCT imaging has been shown to be useful in some types of inflammatory diseases. On EDI-OCT, the choroidal thickness and the choroidal vascularity index (CVI = the ratio between hyper- and hyporeflective spaces measured in the choroidal layer on structural OCT B-scans) were increased compared to controls in eyes with an acute presentation of Vogt-Koyanagi-Harada disease (VKH). In addition, there was loss of focal hyperreflectivity within the inner choroid [57, 58]. Both the choroidal thickness and the CVI also showed a significant reduction in response to treatment [57, 58]; hence, monitoring choroidal thickness may be important in assessing response to treatment and detecting early recurrence in eyes with Vogt-Koyanagi-Harada disease.

Studies of eyes with multiple evanescent white dot syndrome have shown that during the acute phase, subfoveal choroidal thickness measured with OCT in both the affected and fellow eye is thicker than that measured in the convalescent stage [59]. Chronic choroidal changes associated with MFC are characterized by localized thinning of the choroid, occlusion of the choroidal vessels, and localized hyperreflectivity that may represent hyperpigmentation of the choroid (Fig. 6a) [60]. Acute stages of MFC are characterized by the presence of sub-RPE material (inflammatory PEDs), choroidal hyperreflectivity (hypertransmission) below these lesions, ellipsoid zone (EZ) disrup-

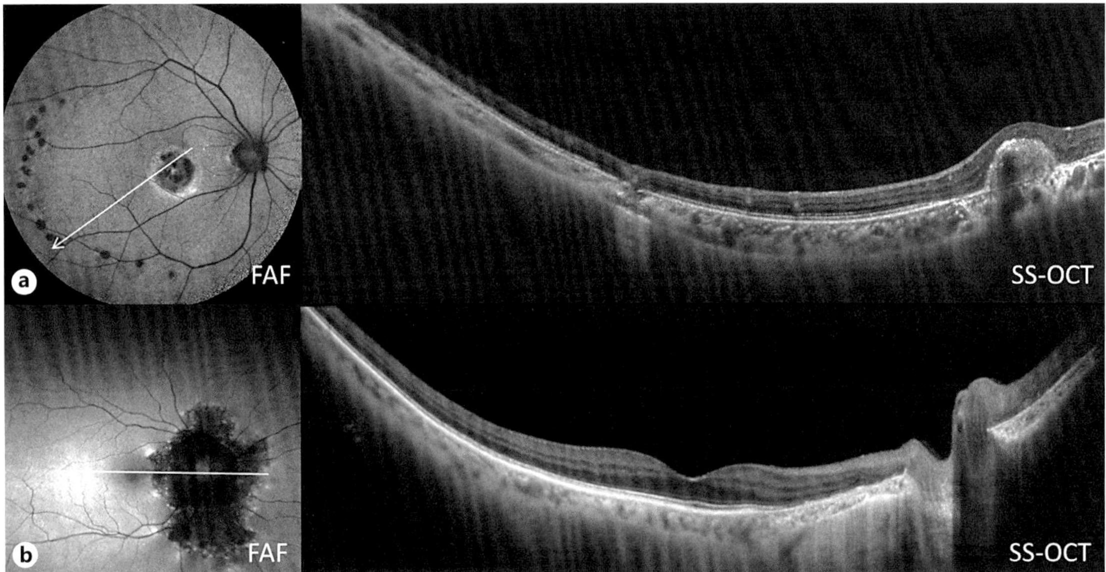

Fig. 6. An example of an eye with multifocal choroiditis (**a**) imaged with fundus autofluorescence (FAF) shows peripheral focal areas of hypoautofluorescent atrophy with subretinal fibrosis at the macula seen as hyperreflective material on optical coherence tomography (OCT). An example of an eye with acute zonal occult outer retinopathy showing the trizonal pattern on FAF and OCT with a zone or normal retina, transition zone, and atrophic zone. SS-OCT, swept-source OCT (**b**).

tion, and overlying vitreous cells [61]. EDI-OCT findings in PIC, often considered a milder form of idiopathic MFC, are similar. In both MCF and PIC, acute changes may evolve into focal areas of outer retinal loss overlying choroidal atrophy corresponding to "punched out" chorioretinal scars seen on clinical examination. Long-term findings associated with chronic disease or multiple recurrences include outer retinal atrophy associated with poor visual acuity and zonal areas of visual field loss. In eyes with birdshot retinochoroiditis, birdshot lesions appear as hyporeflective spaces within the choroid, and choroidal thickness measured on EDI-OCT has been shown to decrease during disease progression [62]. Eyes with acute zonal occult outer retinopathy have been reported to show a trizonal pattern of abnormalities seen on multimodal imaging; zone 1 shows normal FAF and SD-OCT, zone 2 shows speckled hyperautofluorescence corresponding to material seen on

SD-OCT, and zone 3 is characterized by atrophy with hypoautofluorescence and photoreceptor, RPE, and choroidal atrophy seen on SD-OCT (Fig. 6b) [63].

OCT is also useful for detecting complications of inflammatory conditions such as secondary choroidal NV and monitoring response to treatment with intravitreal anti-VEGF therapy [64]. Inflammatory NV is typically type 2 NV, and OCT imaging of the acute lesions may show multiple, distinctive finger-like projections extending from the area of active type 2 NV into the outer retina described as the "pitchfork sign" [65].

OCT and Inherited Retinal Diseases

SD-OCT in inherited retinal diseases including macular dystrophies offers an opportunity to correlate symptoms with depth-resolved struc-

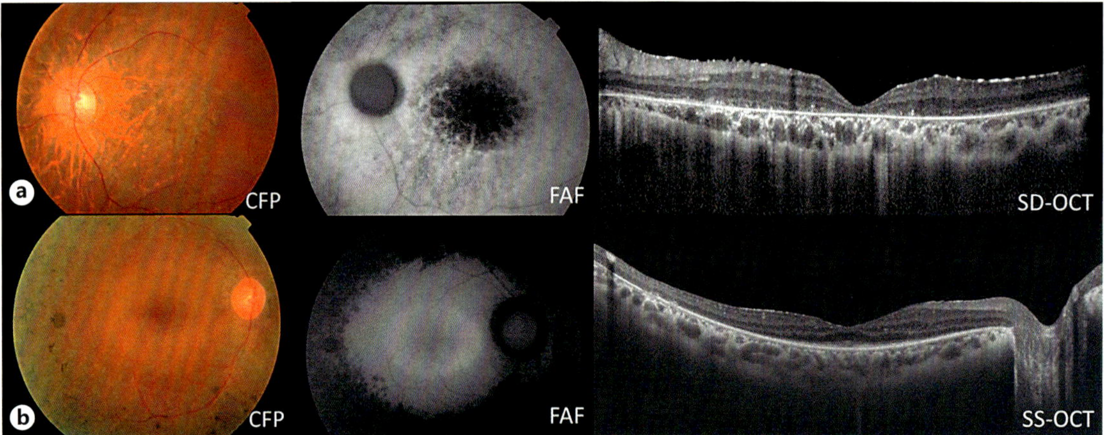

Fig. 7. An example of an eye with cone-rod dystrophy (**a**) that shows that loss of the photoreceptor layers may be complete in the macular region, but preserved in the peripheral regions of the fundus. The central outer retinal loss corresponds to the area of hypoautofluorescence on fundus autofluorescence (FAF). An example of an eye with retinitis pigmentosa (**b**) with a loss of photoreceptor layer that directly corresponds to the inner abnormal FAF border within the central ring. CFP, color fundus photo; SD-OCT, spectral-domain optical coherence tomography; SS-OCT, swept-source OCT.

tural changes in a manner not possible with fundus examination alone. Choroidal OCT imaging can help to confirm a diagnosis and aid in monitoring disease progression. The OCT findings in the most common inherited retinal disease, retinitis pigmentosa, include loss of both photoreceptor layers and retinal nerve fiber layer (Fig. 7b) [66]. The progressive loss of the outer retinal layers can be directly correlated with abnormalities seen on FAF at the posterior border forming a ring corresponding to the visual field boundary (Fig. 7b). In the early stages, the central cone photoreceptors may be spared, and the photoreceptor loss may be patchy, but progression into more complete lesions affecting the entire retina may occur in the later stages with thinning of the RPE-Bruch's membrane complex [67].

OCT findings characteristic of cone dystrophy in the early stages only involve the loss of the interdigitation zone (IZ), with or without foveal cavitation. In the later stages, the photoreceptor layer may be completely lost in the macular re-

gion but preserved in the peripheral fundus. There is also generalized thinning of the RPE layer and choroid (Fig. 7a) [68]. The findings of SD-OCT in eyes with Stargadt's disease include a hyperplastic RPE with hyperreflectivity seen in the fovea region. Irregularity at the fovea in the residual neurosensory retina may make it difficult to distinguish the different photoreceptor layers in the parafoveal region [69]. Hyperreflective spots in the outer retinal layers and the RPE/Bruch's membrane complex are representative of retinal flecks [70]. Overall, OCT imaging allows quantitative, in vivo imaging of the photoreceptor layer and RPE in patients with Stargardt disease and similar macular dystrophies. Choroidal thinning and atrophy can be observed in some cases. SD-OCT shows that most of the crystalline deposits in Bietti retinal dystrophy are located at the level of the RPE/Bruch's membrane complex in portions of the retina that were spared from patchy degeneration [71]. One study with serial imaging showed that the disappearance of the crystals was associated with severe disruption and thinning of the RPE/Bruch's membrane complex [71]. In the outer nuclear layer (ONL), hyperrefractive, spherical structures are associated with areas of ongoing retinal degeneration [72].

SD-OCT allows visualization of changes in the retinal and choroidal structures which can aid in monitoring disease progression in Best vitelliform macular dystrophy [73]. In the previtelliform and vittelliform stages, there is a thickened middle highly reflective layer between the RPE/Bruch's complex and the EZ, with a dome-shaped elevation seen at the fovea due to the accumulation of hyperreflective material. The ONL is thinned both over the contour of the elevation and beyond the margins of the dome. During the pseudohypopyon stage, there is a localized neurosensory retinal detachment with clumps of hyperreflective subretinal material and small hyperreflective mounds observed at the level of the RPE/Bruch's complex, seen at the base of this detachment. At the vitelliruptive stage, greyish tissue is seen in the middle of these lesions, corresponding to 2 types of hyperreflective mounds at the level of the RPE/Bruch's complex. The first type of mound is associated with shadowing of underlying choroidal structures. The second type is associated with collapse of the overlying outer retinal layers and hyperreflectivity of the underlying choroid [73]. At the atrophic stage, there is complete loss of the EZ with thinning of the overlying ONL associated with visual impairment. The RPE/Bruch's membrane complex is relatively well preserved. SD-OCT findings of adult-onset foveomacular dystrophy showing an acquired vitelliform lesion include hyperreflective clumps of vitelliform material within the ONL and outer plexiform layer. The RPE/Bruch's membrane complex is either normal, absent over the vitelliform lesion or becomes thickened and less well defined. One study showed choroidal thickening, RPE mottling and discrete PEDs occurring in adult-onset vitelliform dystrophy, and this was in contrast to choroidal thinning observed in advanced AMD [74]. Some of these findings, including PEDs and thicker choroids, suggest there may be some overlap between the diagnoses of nonfamilial adult-onset acquired vitelliform dystrophy and pachychoroid pigment epitheliopathy.

OCT and Choroidal Tumors

Certain distinctive characteristics seen on OCT can help differentiate various choroidal tumors. In addition, EDI-OCT and SS-OCT, used to image choroidal tumors, may allow depth-resolved delineation of the borders of the tumor, which is useful for monitoring tumor size, malignant transformation, response to therapy and recurrence. EDI-OCT has been shown to be useful in differentiating small choroidal melanomas from choroidal nevi (Fig. 8a). Features of increased lesion thickness, subretinal fluid, subretinal orange pigment deposition, retinal irregularities and shaggy photoreceptors are features suggestive of a choroidal melanoma [75]. For melanotic lesions, SS-OCT shows features such as internal vessels, granularity and cavities [76]. Large choroidal vessels detected on SS-OCT, which border nevi, have been associated with the development of subretinal fluid [76]. SD-OCT imaging of eyes with choroidal osteomas show that the majority of these lesions are isoreflective, with some eyes showing overlying choroidal atrophy and retinal degenerative changes. Vascular tumors like choroidal hemangiomas show a regular sponge-like pattern on EDI-OCT [77] with a characteristic multilobular pattern, and a hyperreflective halo surrounding the tumor seen on en face SS-OCT. Common features of choroidal metastases seen on EDI-OCT, are overlying choriocapillaris thinning, plateau-shaped tumors, shaggy photoreceptors, and subretinal fluid with highly reflective speckles. For the

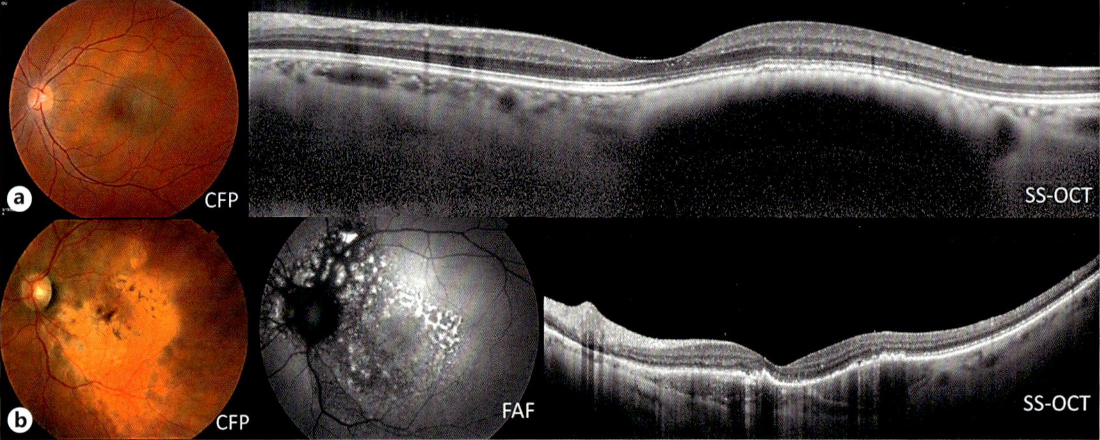

Fig. 8. An eye with a choroidal nevus (**a**) involving the macula. The swept-source optical coherence tomography (SS-OCT) shows choroidal compression at the tumor apex with posterior shadowing. An eye affected by Erdheim-Chester disease shows pigment deposition and infiltrative choroidal masses on SS-OCT (**b**). CFP, color fundus photo; FAF, fundus autofluorescence; SS-OCT, swept-source OCT.

evaluation of small metastatic tumors, EDI-OCT was shown to be more sensitive than ultrasonography. EDI-OCT findings in eyes with primary intraocular lymphoma with choroidal involvement include increased interstitial choroidal thickness when compared to normal controls, and these parameters were significantly reduced in response to treatment [78]. More rarely, ocular involvement of other forms of infiltrative diseases such as Erdheim-Chester disease has been detected also by SS-OCT as choroidal masses (Fig. 8b) [79].

Conclusion

Recent advances in OCT technology including EDI-OCT and SS-OCT have allowed high-resolution choroidal imaging, which have overcome many of the prior challenges associated with the posterior location of the choroid and light attenuation from the RPE and retinal structures [3]. The ability to correlate in vivo choroidal findings, overlying RPE and photoreceptor changes, and visual function is useful for diagnosis and management of a wide range of choroidal diseases.

References

1 Yannuzzi LA: Indocyanine green angiography: a perspective on use in the clinical setting. Am J Ophthalmol 2011; 151:745–751.e741.

2 Inoue R, Sawa M, Tsujikawa M, Gomi F: Association between the efficacy of photodynamic therapy and indocyanine green angiography findings for central serous chorioretinopathy. Am J Ophthalmol 2010;149:441–446.e441–442.

3 Regatieri CV, Branchini L, Fujimoto JG, Duker JS: Choroidal imaging using spectral-domain optical coherence tomography. Retina 2012;32:865–876.

4 Rosenfeld PJ: Optical coherence tomography and the development of antiangiogenic therapies in neovascular age-related macular degeneration. Invest Ophthalmol Vis Sci 2016;57:OCT14–OCT26.

5 Spaide RF, Koizumi H, Pozzoni MC: Enhanced depth imaging spectral-domain optical coherence tomography. Am J Ophthalmol 2008;146:496–500.

6 Spaide RF: Enhanced depth imaging optical coherence tomography of retinal pigment epithelial detachment in age-related macular degeneration. Am J Ophthalmol 2009;147:644–652.

7 Spaide RF: Disease expression in non-exudative age-related macular degeneration varies with choroidal thickness. Retina, Epub ahead of print.

8 Mazaraki K, Fassnacht-Riederle H, Blum R, Becker M, Michels S: Change in choroidal thickness after intravitreal aflibercept in pretreated and treatment-naive eyes for neovascular age-related macular degeneration. Br J Ophthalmol 2015;99:1341–1344.

9 Gupta P, Ting DS, Thakku SG, et al: Detailed characterization of choroidal morphologic and vascular features in age-related macular degeneration and polypoidal choroidal vasculopathy. Retina 2017;37:2269–2280.

10 Ng DS, Cheung CY, Luk FO, et al: Advances of optical coherence tomography in myopia and pathologic myopia. Eye (Lond) 2016;30:901–916.

11 Shields CL, Mashayekhi A, Materin MA, et al: Optical coherence tomography of choroidal nevus in 120 patients. Retina 2005;25:243–252.

12 Dolz-Marco R, Litts KM, Tan ACS, Freund KB, Curcio CA: The evolution of outer retinal tubulation, a neurodegeneration and gliosis prominent in macular diseases. Ophthalmology 2017;124: 1353–1367.

13 Tan ACS, Astroz P, Dansingani KK, et al: The evolution of the plateau, an optical coherence tomography signature seen in geographic atrophy. Invest Ophthalmol Vis Sci 2017;58:2349–2358.

14 Copete S, Flores-Moreno I, Montero JA, Duker JS, Ruiz-Moreno JM: Direct comparison of spectral-domain and swept-source OCT in the measurement of choroidal thickness in normal eyes. Br J Ophthal 2014;98:334–338.

15 Philip AM, Gerendas BS, Zhang L, et al: Choroidal thickness maps from spectral domain and swept source optical coherence tomography: algorithmic versus ground truth annotation. Br J Ophthalmol 2016;100:1372–1376.

16 Margolis R, Spaide RF: A pilot study of enhanced depth imaging optical coherence tomography of the choroid in normal eyes. Am J Ophthalmol 2009;147: 811–815.

17 Lee GY, Yu S, Kang HG, Kim JS, Lee KW, Lee JH: Choroidal thickness variation according to refractive error measured by spectral domain-optical coherence tomography in Korean children. Korean J Ophthalmol 2017;31:151–158.

18 Tan AC, Simhaee D, Balaratnasingam C, Dansingani KK, Yannuzzi LA: A perspective on the nature and frequency of pigment epithelial detachments. Am J Ophthalmol 2016;172:13–27.

19 Bird AC, Bressler NM, Bressler SB, et al: An international classification and grading system for age-related maculopathy and age-related macular degeneration. The International ARM Epidemiological Study Group. Surv Ophthalmol 1995;39: 367–374.

20 Kim SW, Oh J, Kwon SS, Yoo J, Huh K: Comparison of choroidal thickness among patients with healthy eyes, early age-related maculopathy, neovascular age-related macular degeneration, central serous chorioretinopathy, and polypoidal choroidal vasculopathy. Retina 2011;31:1904–1911.

21 Mrejen S, Spaide RF: The relationship between pseudodrusen and choroidal thickness. Retina 2014;34:1560–1566.

22 Mrejen-Uretsky S, Ayrault S, Nghiem-Buffet S, Quentel G, Cohen SY: Choroidal thickening in patients with cuticular drusen combined with vitelliform macular detachment. Retina 2016;36:1111–1118.

23 Esmaeelpour M, Ansari-Shahrezaei S, Glittenberg C, et al: Choroid, Haller's, and Sattler's layer thickness in intermediate age-related macular degeneration with and without fellow neovascular eyes. Invest Ophthalmol Vis Sci 2014;55: 5074–5080.

24 Balaratnasingam C, Yannuzzi LA, Querques G, Curcio CA, Capuano V, Dansingani KK, Jung JJ, Souied E, Naysan J, Freund KB: Associations between retinal pigment epithelium and drusen volume changes during the lifecycle of large drusenoid pigment epithelial detachments. Invest Ophthalmol Vis Sci 2016; 57:5479–5489.

25 Capuano V, Souied EH, Miere A, Jung C, Costanzo E, Querques G: Choroidal maps in non-exudative age-related macular degeneration. Br J Ophthalmol 2016;100:677–682.

26 Dolz-Marco R, Gal-Or O, Freund KB: Choroidal thickness influences near-infrared reflectance intensity in eyes with geographic atrophy due to age-related macular degeneration. Invest Ophthalmol Vis Sci 2016;57:6440–6446.

27 Lee JY, Lee DH, Lee JY, Yoon YH: Correlation between subfoveal choroidal thickness and the severity or progression of nonexudative age-related macular degeneration. Invest Ophthalmol Vis Sci 2013;54:7812–7818.

28 Pilotto E, Guidolin F, Convento E, et al: En face optical coherence tomography to detect and measure geographic atrophy. Invest Ophthalmol Vis Sci 2015;56: 8120–8124.

29 Freund KB, Zweifel SA, Engelbert M: Do we need a new classification for choroidal neovascularization in age-related macular degeneration? Retina 2010;30: 1333–1349.

30 Mrejen S, Sarraf D, Mukkamala SK, Freund KB: Multimodal imaging of pigment epithelial detachment: a guide to evaluation. Retina 2013;33:1735–1762.

31 Hernandez-Martinez P, Dolz-Marco R, Hervas-Marin D, Andreu-Fenoll M, Gallego-Pinazo R, Arevalo JF: Choroidal thickness and visual prognosis in type 1 lesion due to neovascular age-related macular degeneration. Eur J Ophthalmol 2017;27:196–200.

32 Dansingani KK, Tan AC, Gilani F, et al: Subretinal hyperreflective material imaged with optical coherence tomography angiography. Am J Ophthalmol 2016; 169:235–248.

33 Malamos P, Sacu S, Georgopoulos M, Kiss C, Pruente C, Schmidt-Erfurth U: Correlation of high-definition optical coherence tomography and fluorescein angiography imaging in neovascular macular degeneration. Invest Ophthalmol Vis Sci 2009;50:4926–4933.

34 Nagiel A, Sarraf D, Sadda SR, et al: Type 3 neovascularization: evolution, association with pigment epithelial detachment, and treatment response as revealed by spectral domain optical coherence tomography. Retina 2015;35: 638–647.

35 Querques G, Souied EH, Freund KB: Multimodal imaging of early stage 1 type 3 neovascularization with simultaneous eye-tracked spectral-domain optical coherence tomography and high-speed real-time angiography. Retina 2013;33:1881–1887.

36 Kim JH, Kim JR, Kang SW, Kim SJ, Ha HS: Thinner choroid and greater drusen extent in retinal angiomatous proliferation than in typical exudative age-related macular degeneration. Am J Ophthalmol 2013;155:743–749, 749.e741–e742.

37 Group CR, Martin DF, Maguire MG, et al: Ranibizumab and bevacizumab for neovascular age-related macular degeneration. N Engl J Med 2011;364:1897–1908.

38 Razavi S, Souied EH, Darvizeh F, Querques G: Assessment of choroidal topographic changes by swept-source optical coherence tomography after intravitreal ranibizumab for exudative age-related macular degeneration. Am J Ophthalmol 2015;160:1006–1013.

39 Dansingani KK, Balaratnasingam C, Naysan J, Freund KB: En face imaging of pachychoroid spectrum disorders with SWEPT-source optical coherence tomography. Retina 2016;36:499–516.

40 Yanagi Y, Ting DSW, Ng WY, et al: Choroidal vascular hyperpermeability as a predictor of treatment response for polypoidal choroidal vasculopathy. Retina, Epub ahead of print.

41 Wong CW, Yanagi Y, Lee WK, et al: Age-related macular degeneration and polypoidal choroidal vasculopathy in Asians. Prog Retin Eye Res 2016;53: 107–139.

42 Tan ACS, Yzer S, Freund KB, Dansingani KK, Phasukkijwatana N, Sarraf D: Choroidal changes associated with serous macular detachment in eyes with staphyloma, dome-shaped macula or tilted disk syndrome. Retina 2017;37: 1544–1554.

43 Gupta P, Jing T, Marziliano P, et al: Distribution and determinants of choroidal thickness and volume using automated segmentation software in a population-based study. Am J Ophthalmol 2015; 159:293–301.e293.

44 Summers JA. The choroid as a sclera growth regulator. Exp Eye Res 2013;114: 120–127.

45 Moriyama M, Ohno-Matsui K, Futagami S, et al: Morphology and long-term changes of choroidal vascular structure in highly myopic eyes with and without posterior staphyloma. Ophthalmology 2007;114:1755–1762.

46 Ohno-Matsui K, Akiba M, Modegi T, et al: Association between shape of sclera and myopic retinochoroidal lesions in patients with pathologic myopia. Invest Ophthalmol Vis Sci 2012;53:6046–6061.

47 Zaben A, Zapata MA, Garcia-Arumi J: Retinal sensitivity and choroidal thickness in high myopia. Retina 2015;35: 398–406.

48 Tan AC, Teo K, Guan OS, Koh A: Long-term outcomes of myopic choroidal neovascularisation treated with combined ranibizumab and dexamethasone characterised by multi-modal imaging. Graefes Arch Clin Exp Ophthalmol 2016;254:1881–1888.

49 Chhablani J, Deepa MJ, Tyagi M, Narayanan R, Kozak I: Fluorescein angiography and optical coherence tomography in myopic choroidal neovascularization. Eye (Lond) 2015;29:519–524.

50 Wong TY, Ohno-Matsui K, Leveziel N, et al: Myopic choroidal neovascularisation: current concepts and update on clinical management. Br J Ophthalmol 2015;99:289–296.

51 Ng WY, Ting DS, Agrawal R, et al: Choroidal structural changes in myopic choroidal neovascularization after treatment with antivascular endothelial growth factor over 1 year. Invest Ophthalmol Vis Sci 2016;57:4933–4939.

52 Ikuno Y, Ohno-Matsui K, Wong TY, et al: Intravitreal aflibercept injection in patients with myopic choroidal neovascularization: the MYRROR study. Ophthalmology 2015;122:1220–1227.

53 Spaide RF, Akiba M, Ohno-Matsui K: Evaluation of peripapillary intrachoroidal cavitation with swept source and enhanced depth imaging optical coherence tomography. Retina 2012;32:1037–1044.

54 Ohno-Matsui K, Akiba M, Moriyama M, Ishibashi T, Hirakata A, Tokoro T: Intrachoroidal cavitation in macular area of eyes with pathologic myopia. Am J Ophthalmol 2012;154:382–393.

55 Imamura Y, Iida T, Maruko I, Zweifel SA, Spaide RF: Enhanced depth imaging optical coherence tomography of the sclera in dome-shaped macula. Am J Ophthalmol 2011;151:297–302.

56 Caillaux V, Gaucher D, Gualino V, Massin P, Tadayoni R, Gaudric A: Morphologic characterization of dome-shaped macula in myopic eyes with serous macular detachment. Am J Ophthalmol 2013;156:958–967.e951.

57 Fong AH, Li KK, Wong D: Choroidal evaluation using enhanced depth imaging spectral-domain optical coherence tomography in Vogt-Koyanagi-Harada disease. Retina 2011;31:502–509.

58 Agrawal R, Li LK, Nakhate V, Khandelwal N, Mahendradas P: Choroidal vascularity index in Vogt-Koyanagi-Harada disease: an EDI-OCT derived tool for monitoring disease progression. Transl Vis Sci Technol 2016;5:7.

59 Aoyagi R, Hayashi T, Masai A, et al: Subfoveal choroidal thickness in multiple evanescent white dot syndrome. Clin Exp Optom 2012;95:212–217.

60 Yasuno Y, Okamoto F, Kawana K, Yatagai T, Oshika T: Investigation of multifocal choroiditis with panuveitis by three-dimensional high-penetration optical coherence tomography. J Biophotonics 2009;2:435–441.

61 Vance SK, Khan S, Klancnik JM, Freund KB: Characteristic spectral-domain optical coherence tomography findings of multifocal choroiditis. Retina 2011;31: 717–723.

62 Boni C, Thorne JE, Spaide RF, et al: Choroidal findings in eyes with birdshot chorioretinitis using enhanced-depth optical coherence tomography. Invest Ophthalmol Vis Sci 2016;57:OCT591–OCT599.

63 Mrejen S, Khan S, Gallego-Pinazo R, Jampol LM, Yannuzzi LA: Acute zonal occult outer retinopathy: a classification based on multimodal imaging. JAMA Ophthalmol 2014;132:1089–1098.

64 Mansour AM, Arevalo JF, Ziemssen F, et al: Long-term visual outcomes of intravitreal bevacizumab in inflammatory ocular neovascularization. Am J Ophthalmol 2009;148:310–316.e312.

65 Hoang QV, Cunningham ET Jr, Sorenson JA, Freund KB: The "pitchfork sign" a distinctive optical coherence tomography finding in inflammatory choroidal neovascularization. Retina 2013;33: 1049–1055.

66 Triolo G, Pierro L, Parodi MB, et al: Spectral domain optical coherence tomography findings in patients with retinitis pigmentosa. Ophthalmic Res 2013; 50:160–164.

67 Oishi A, Ogino K, Nakagawa S, et al: Longitudinal analysis of the peripapillary retinal nerve fiber layer thinning in patients with retinitis pigmentosa. Eye 2013;27:597–604.

68 Inui E, Oishi A, Oishi M, et al: Tomographic comparison of cone-rod and rod-cone retinal dystrophies. Graefes Arch Clin Exp Ophthalmol 2014;252: 1065–1069.

69 Saxena S, Mishra N, Meyer CH: Three-dimensional spectral domain optical coherence tomography in Stargardt disease and fundus flavimaculatus. J Ocul Biol Dis Infor 2012;5:13–18.

70 Querques G, Prato R, Coscas G, Soubrane G, Souied EH: In vivo visualization of photoreceptor layer and lipofuscin accumulation in Stargardt's disease and fundus flavimaculatus by high resolution spectral-domain optical coherence tomography. Clin Ophthalmol 2009;3:693–699.

71 Halford S, Liew G, Mackay DS, et al: Detailed phenotypic and genotypic characterization of Bietti crystalline dystrophy. Ophthalmology 2014;121:1174–1184.

72 Kojima H, Otani A, Ogino K, et al: Outer retinal circular structures in patients with Bietti crystalline retinopathy. Br J Ophthalmol 2012;96:390–393.

73 Ferrara DC, Costa RA, Tsang S, Calucci D, Jorge R, Freund KB: Multimodal fundus imaging in Best vitelliform macular dystrophy. Graefes Arch Clin Exp Ophthalmol 2010;248:1377–1386.

74 Coscas F, Puche N, Coscas G, et al: Comparison of macular choroidal thickness in adult onset foveomacular vitelliform dystrophy and age-related macular degeneration. Invest Ophthalmol Vis Sci 2014;55:64–69.

75 Shields CL, Kaliki S, Rojanaporn D, Ferenczy SR, Shields JA: Enhanced depth imaging optical coherence tomography of small choroidal melanoma: comparison with choroidal nevus. Arch Ophthalmol 2012;130:850–856.

76 Francis JH, Pang CE, Abramson DH, et al: Swept-source optical coherence tomography features of choroidal nevi. Am J Ophthalmol 2015;159:169–176.e161.

77 Filloy A, Caminal JM, Arias L, Jordan S, Catala J: Swept source optical coherence tomography imaging of a series of choroidal tumours. Can J Ophthalmol 2015;50:242–248.

78 Egawa M, Mitamura Y, Sano H, et al: Changes of choroidal structure after treatment for primary intraocular lymphoma: retrospective, observational case series. BMC Ophthalmol 2015;15:136.

79 Tan ACS, Yzer S, Atebara N, Marr BP, Verdijk RM, Dalm VASH, Freund KB, Yannuzzi L, Missotten T: Three cases of erdheim-chester disease with intraocular manifestations: imaging and histopathology findings of a rare entity. Am J Ophthalmol 2017;176:141–147.

Anna C.S. Tan
Singapore National Eye Center
11 Third Hospital Avenue
Singapore 168751 (Singapore)
E-Mail annacstan@gmail.com

Cunha-Vaz J, Koh A (eds): Imaging Techniques.
ESASO Course Series. Basel, Karger, 2018, vol 10, pp 52–64 (DOI: 10.1159/000487412)

Optical Coherence Tomography Angiography

Giuseppe Querques[a] · Riccardo Sacconi[a, b] · Adriano Carnevali[a, c] ·
Lea Querques[a] · Ilaria Zucchiatti[a] · Francesco Bandello[a]

[a]Department of Ophthalmology, University Vita-Salute, IRCCS Ospedale San Raffaele, Milan, [b]Eye Clinic, Department of
Neurological, Biomedical and Movement Sciences, University of Verona, Verona, and [c]Department of Ophthalmology,
University of "Magna Graecia," Catanzaro, Italy

Abstract

Optical coherence tomography angiography (OCT-A) is
a new tool able to visualize the different retinal plexuses
and choroidal plexus, and it is a dye-free, rapid, and
three-dimensional method. A new era in retinal imaging
has begun, and retinal specialists have to deal with this
novel diagnostic tool. However, OCT-A is a very recent
technology and, as such, its clinical applications have still
to be determined. For these reasons, dye angiographies
(fluorescein angiography and indocyanine green angiography) are still the current gold standard to study the
retinal and choroidal vessels. In this chapter, we focus on
current OCT-A applications in several retinal diseases
(age-related macular degeneration, diabetic retinopathy, and pachychoroid pigment epitheliopathy), and discuss how this new technology could revolutionize our
daily clinical practice.   © 2018 S. Karger AG, Basel

Fluorescein angiography (FA) and indocyanine
green angiography (ICGA) are the current gold
standard to study the retinal and choroidal vessels, respectively; however, both tests are invasive
and associated with potentially life-threatening
side effects (nausea and rarely anaphylaxis) [1, 2].
Leakage of dye in the later frames of the angiographic examinations is used to identify any inju-
ries like retinal vascular abnormalities or choroidal neovascularization (CNV).

Optical coherence tomography angiography
(OCT-A) is a new method to visualize the different retinal plexuses and choroidal plexus, and it is
a dye-free, rapid, and three-dimensional method.
OCT-A is based on algorithms that convert multiple A-scans to OCT-A images. OCT angiograms
are coregistered with OCT B-scans that are ob-

tained concurrently, allowing for visualization of both retinal flow and structure in tandem. Images are based on the concept that in a static eye the only moving structure in the fundus of the eye is blood flowing through vessels, and the contrast is generated based on the difference between moving cells in the vasculature and the surrounding static tissue. OCT-A and FA provide different morphostructural data. The information generated by combining these two diagnostic tools could permit to go deeper into the pathophysiology of chorioretinal and optic nerve diseases, and, thus, to set the foundations to improve everyday clinical practice [3].

A new era in retinal imaging has begun, and retinal specialists have to deal with this novel diagnostic tool [3]. However, OCT-A is a very recent technology and, as such, its clinical applications have still to be determined. Comparative studies between OCT-A and FA across the wide spectrum of retinal pathologies are warranted in order to better understand information obtained through OCT-A. Technological advances will surely overcome some methodological limitations, including motion artifacts, segmentation errors, projection artifacts, and suboptimal resolution for small-caliber vessels due to signal averaging.

We report current OCT-A applications and discuss how this new technology could revolutionize our daily clinical practice.

Different Devices Using Different Algorithms

The OCT-A technology is based on different types of algorithm such as split-spectrum amplitude-decorrelation angiography (SSADA), optical microangiography (OMAG), OCT-A ratio analysis (OCTARA), or full-spectrum amplitude-decorrelation angiography (FSADA).

The Optovue AngioVue system (Optovue Inc., Freemont, CA, USA) is a spectral-domain OCT (SD-OCT) that generates OCT-A images using the SSADA algorithm. The instrument has an A-scan rate of 70,000 scans per second, and each OCT-A volume contains 304 × 304 A-scans with two consecutive B-scans captured at each fixed position. The SSADA algorithm extracts the OCT-A information. It detects motion in blood vessel lumen by measuring variations in reflected OCT signal amplitude between consecutive cross-sectional scans. Two orthogonal OCT-A volumes are acquired for orthogonal registration using motion correction technology to minimize motion artifacts arising from fixation changes [4–6].

Zeiss HD-OCT Cirrus 5000 with Angioplex OCT-A (Zeiss Meditech Inc., Dublin, CA, USA) is an SD-OCT that generates OCT-A images using the OMAG algorithm. The instrument has an A-scan rate of 68,000 scans per second and an axial resolution of 5 μm in tissue and a transverse resolution of 15 μm [7]. The standard scanning patterns available on Zeiss HD-OCT Cirrus 5000 with Angioplex are 3 × 3 and 6 × 6 mm, but also 9 × 9 images could be generated. Each 3 × 3 image contains 245 A-scan in each B-scan, repeated four times in the same position. Each 6 × 6 image contains 350 A-scan in each B-scan, repeated two times in the same position. The angiographic images are generated using the OMAG algorithm that analyzes differences in both intensity and phase information from repeated B-scans at the same position. Zeiss Angioplex OCT-A also incorporates FastTrac technology to reduce movement artifacts.

The DRI OCT imaging system (Topcon, Tokyo, Japan) is a swept-source OCT technology that generates OCT-A images using the OCTARA algorithm. The instrument can acquire 100,000 A-scans per second over a 3 × 3 mm area that could be enlarged to 6 × 6 mm (Triton and Atlantis) or even to 12 × 9 mm (Atlantis). OCTRA aims to provide improved detection sensitivity of low blood flow and reduced motion artifacts without compromising axial resolution [8].

The Spectralis OCT2 device (Heidelberg Engineering, Heidelberg, Germany) is an SD-OCT that is able to acquire 85,000 A-scans per second.

The FSADA algorithm guarantees clear differentiation between blood flow and static tissue without sacrificing axial resolution in OCT imaging [9]. The number of B-scans changes in relation to the volume scan acquired. Furthermore, the use of an active eye-tracking system (TrueTrack, Heidelberg Engineering, Heidelberg, Germany) enables the acquisition of very reliable OCT volume scans without motion artifacts.

OCT-A Analysis, Segmentations, and Artifacts

Dye angiographies (FA and ICGA) have several limitations to detect the different retinal and choroidal plexuses. Although FA and ICGA could be useful in the study of retinal or choroidal circulation, they play a limited role in the study of the retinal deep capillary plexus (DCP) and of the choriocapillaris due to the absence of depth resolution, the limited spatial resolution, and the obfuscation of vascular details because of dye leakage [10–12].

OCT-A is a new technique that provides unprecedented clues to the state of retinal vascular flow in a depth-resolved manner thanks to the possibility to visualize the vascular networks in separate layers. However, OCT-A examinations need careful axial segmentation in order to preserve important data on perfused structures and to avoid the risk of generation of superimposed images [13]. An automated segmentation algorithm for both retinal and choroidal layers is typically provided by the majority of different OCT-A devices. This algorithm is able to detect several different retinal layers, from the inner limiting membrane to the retinal pigment epithelium (RPE). Automated layer segmentation is useful in the clinical practice to provide an extremely fast way to delineate the presence of a decorrelation signal due to perfused vascular structures in each OCT-A image. Typically, all OCT-A software reports the segmentation of the superficial capillary plexus (SCP) and DCP taken at the reported exact

histological site. In fact, histological findings allocate the retinal SCP to the ganglion cell layer, and the DCP to the inner nuclear layer. Using OCT-A, the SCP is located between the internal limiting membrane and the posterior part of the inner plexiform layer, while the DCP is situated in the inner nuclear layer. Furthermore, OCT-A software also reports the segmentation of the choriocapillaris and of the choroid.

Although automated segmentation allows prompt analysis of different vascular layers, it can suffer from segmentation errors, especially in case of accentuated macular abnormalities. In these cases, specific manual correction allows one to modify the shape and the localization of each layer.

Furthermore, it is important to consider that OCT-A images could be affected by projection artifacts. These occur from superficial retinal vessels, which can be seen in deeper retinal layers, or from retinal and choroidal vessels, which can be seen in scleral tissue. These projection artifacts are almost always present and are visible in any layer that is located below the perfused vasculature.

OCT-A in the Clinical Practice

Age-Related Macular Degeneration
Age-related macular degeneration (AMD) is the leading cause of severe visual impairment in older adults in all countries. Neovascular AMD is responsible for severe vison loss in 90% of AMD cases. OCT-A enables a better morphological classification of different neovascular lesions characterizing AMD.

In 2013, Querques et al. [14] first described treatment-naïve quiescent CNV in intermediate AMD [15]. FA reveals treatment-naïve quiescent CNV consisting of ill-defined hyperfluorescent lesion showing no leakage or pooling of dye in the late angiographic frames, and it is similar to type 1 CNV as described by Gass [16]. In ICGA, quiescent CNV appears as a hyperfluorescent vascu-

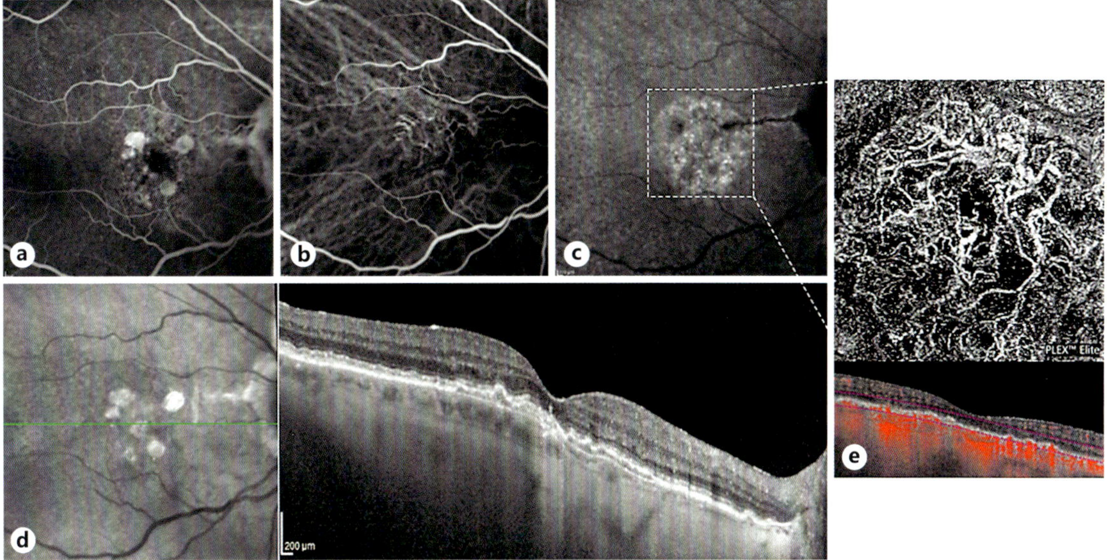

Fig. 1. Multimodal imaging of a patient affected by quiescent type 1 CNV. **a** FA showing inhomogeneous small hyperfluorescence without leakage. **b**, **c** Early and late phases of ICGA showing late plaque which corresponds to the quiescent CNV. **d** Combined infrared and structural OCT B-scan passing through the fovea showing the presence of a flat irregular elevation of the RPE with moderately reflective material in the sub-RPE space, compatible with type 1 CNV. **e** 3 × 3 mm OCT-A obtained using ORCC slab (outer retina-choroidal capillaries) and corresponding OCT B-scan showing the quiescent CNV.

lar network in the early to intermediate frames and has the appearance of a hyperfluorescent plaque in the late angiographic frames [14]. With SD-OCT, quiescent CNV appears as an irregular elevation of the RPE, with its major axis in the horizontal plane (width/height ratio >1). This irregular pigment epithelium detachment (PED) exhibits moderate reflectivity in the sub-RPE space, and the hyperreflective Bruch's membrane (BM) is clearly visible. The absence of subretinal or intraretinal exudation in repeated SD-OCT for at least 6 months is essential if CNV is to be classified as quiescent [14].

In 2016, Carnevali et al. [17] observed that OCT-A was able to identify treatment-naïve quiescent CNV in intermediate AMD, with good levels of sensitivity and specificity compared with invasive imaging techniques, based on OCT-A classification. OCT-A is able to identify microvascular structures and can be used to assess the morphol-

ogy of type 1 neovascularization. OCT-A visualizes the retinal vasculature by detecting intravascular blood flow. Quiescent CNVs may be visualized by means of OCT-A in great details characterized by their size, morphology, blood vessel caliper and presence of subretinal fluid [18] (Fig. 1).

Type 1 neovascularization arises from the choriocapillaris and develops under the RPE. OCT-A enables more accurate identification of type 1 lesions compared to traditional FA [19]. While FA can identify the superficial retinal capillary plexus, OCT-A poorly visualizes the deep retinal capillary plexus and the choroid. PED may demonstrate pooling or stippled fluorescence with FA, but the identification of the causative neovascular complex is very challenging and only minimally improved with ICGA. Conversely, OCT-A utilizes amplitude or phase decorrelation technology with high-frequency and dense volumetric scanning to detect red blood cell movement and to visualize blood vessels at various depth-resolved levels of the retina and choroid. OCT-A of type 1 neovascularization has led to a detailed assessment of the microvascular morphologies of these vessel complexes, which are typically hidden under a PED. Recent studies have identified the different morphologies of these neovascular lesions and have applied varying descriptive terms to label these structures, which are best visualized with OCT-A. These labels include "umbrella vessels," "seafan and medusa vessels," "tangled network pattern," and "pruned vascular and blossoming tree." When imaged with OCT-A in the acute phase, the neovascularization has the appearance of a tangled web of fine vessels [20, 21]. Chronic type 1 lesions have shown a distinctly different morphology. In a large study using OCT-A to describe chronic type 1 lesions previously treated with multiple intravitreal anti-VEGF injections, Kuehlewein et al. [22] analyzed 33 eyes with AMD and PED associated with type 1 lesions that were large and mature; these averaged 5.79 mm^2 in area. Of note, 75% of the cases showed a highly organized vascular complex with vessels branching from a core trunk and multiple large, dilated feeder vessels. OCT-A has also been employed to study the late fibrotic stage of type 1 neovascularization in AMD. Miere et al. [21] analyzed 49 eyes diagnosed with subretinal fibrosis complicating neovascular AMD, 39 of which were either type 1 or combined type 1 and type 2 lesions. Additionally, OCT-A has been utilized to characterize the response of type 1 neovascularization to antiangiogenic therapy. Muakkassa et al. [23] studied 6 patients with treatment-naïve CNV, 4 of which had type 1 lesions. Eyes were scanned before anti-VEGF treatment and at follow-up visits in order to assess the area of each neovascular lesion and its greatest linear dimension. Despite great advancements in the identification and analysis of type 1 CNV with OCT-A, considerable limitations still exist. Since split-

spectrum amplitude-decorrelation technology relies on the detection of erythrocyte movement, any movement of a patient's head or eyes during image acquisition results in significant artifact production and decreased image quality [20–24]. In addition, the generation of projection artifacts and the shadowing of the SCP onto the deeper layers of the retina can make it difficult to distinguish normal vessels from pathologic OCT-A of type 1 CNV in AMD.

More advanced software able to remove or correct for these types of artifacts will greatly improve the utility of OCT-A in clinical practice. Furthermore, increased precision and the ability to easily modify slab segmentation for follow-up encounters is also necessary in order to more accurately evaluate changes in vessel complexes over time and following anti-VEGF therapy.

OCT-A continues to be a promising method for identifying the morphology and monitoring the treatment response of type 1 neovascularization and PED, as conventional angiography cannot adequately visualize occult pathologic vessels [12]. The ability to identify neovascular complexes and their distinct microvascular structures via OCT-A empowers the retinologist to directly gauge and measure the response of pathologic vessels to intravitreal anti-VEGF therapy or other novel therapeutic agents. Qualitative assessment of morphological changes in a vessel complex in response to therapy may be valuable. Important quantitative measurements include baseline and follow-up lesion area, lesion vessel density, and greatest linear dimension. This type of qualitative and quantitative OCT-A analysis performed on a larger scale may be used to better assess the efficacy of anti-VEGF treatment in research trials, leading to more efficacious pharmacotherapeutics, and in the clinical area, leading to more optimal care for patients with neovascular AMD [19].

Well-defined CNV, or type 2 CNV, also called classic CNV or preepithelial CNV, is the least representative phenotype of exudative AMD, accounting for 17.6% of all neovascular AMD cases [25]. To date, FA remains the gold standard for imaging AMD at initial presentation if neovascular complications are anticipated. Type 2 CNV presents a well-demarcated area of hyperfluorescence (corresponding to the neovascular membrane) in the early frames of an angiogram. Late phases are marked by a progressive leakage of dye from this area [26]. Type 2 CNV can be visualized using OCT-A with very typical patterns. The neovascular membrane appears either as a medusa-shaped complex or a glomerulus-shaped lesion in the outer retina [27]. The medusa-shaped complex is characterized by a well-defined oval shape, generally formed by a very dense high-flow network at diagnosis because of the high activity of this kind of CNV. The glomerulus-shaped lesion is rounded, well defined, and full of a very dense maze of small new vessels. No vascular abnormality is detected in either the superficial or deep retinal capillary layers. Two automatic segmentations on OCT-A are interesting for type 2 CNV secondary to AMD. The first, called the "outer retina," is delimited between the inner nuclear layer and BM, and the second, called the "choriocapillaris layer" is located under BM. At the pathophysiologic level, type 2 CNV involves choroidal new vessels that cross BM and grow up above the neurosensory retina. This feature allows us to visualize these lesions on the outer retina. One or more central feeder vessels that expand in radial branches and continue deeply into the more profound choroidal layers are visible. In a short series, the feeder vessel was identified in 9 cases out of 14 [27]. It is exceptional to distinguish and recognize the afferent of the efferent branches.

The complex morphology of type 2 CNV changes after treatment using vascular endothelial growth factor antagonists, leading to a decrease in size and density, and the prominent tangle becomes less compact. After long-term treatment, the neovascular lesion becomes fibrotic and its appearance on OCT-A changes [21].

Analysis of OCT-A images may be subjected to many artifacts, like projection artifacts, which can lead to misinterpretation, and the detection of such artifacts requires a clinician to perform an interactive evaluation [28]. Conversely, this new technology allows such great resolution of vascular layers that we can colorize each one and overlap them.

By definition, type 2 CNV is preepithelial, so any vessel in this area ("outer retina") can be considered type 2 CNV and abnormal.

Identification of type 2 CNV appears easily feasible for any clinician using OCT-A, especially in areas where there are normally no vessels, like in the subretinal space, if the interpretation rules are respected [28].

Origin, anatomic location, and imaging characteristics are still controversial for type 3 neovascularization. In 2008, Freund et al. [29] described type 3 neovascularization as two previously described lesions: retinal angiomatous proliferation and chorioretinal anastomosis [30, 31]. Yannuzzi et al. [30, 32] described retinal angiomatous proliferations as a distinct form of neovascular AMD consisting of focal neovascular proliferation from the deep retinal layer extending into the subretinal space and possibly communicating with a CNV. Commonly, they are described as a hyperfluorescent intraretinal vascular complex characterized by retinal-retinal anastomosis on FA determining a hot spot on ICGA late frames.

OCT-A allows blood flow visualization enabling a detailed imaging of the retinal microcirculation and could become a gold standard for the detection, diagnosis, and follow-up of these intraretinal lesions.

On OCT-A, type 3 neovascularization can be defined as a retinal-retinal anastomosis that rises from the DCP, determining high-flow, tuft-shaped neovascular lesion in the segmentation corresponding to the outer retinal layers, finally

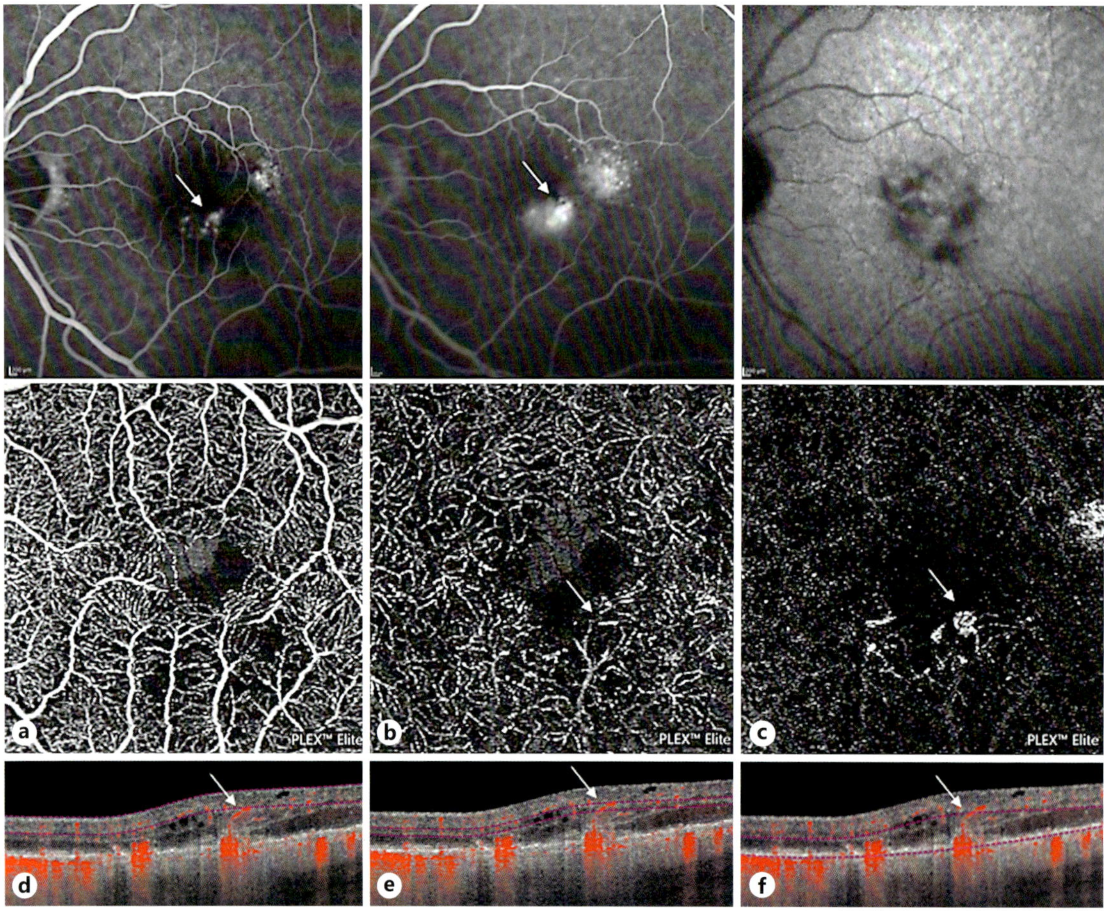

Fig. 2. Multimodal imaging of a patient affected by type 3 CNV. Early and late phases of FA (**a**, **b**) and ICGA (**c**) showing a hyperfluorescent lesion characterized by leakage. 3 × 3 mm OCT-A images and corresponding OCT B-scan showing no abnormalities of the SCP (**d**), but a lesion with flow in the DCP (**e**) and ORCC slab (**f**).

abutting in the sub-RPE space (Fig. 2). In the choriocapillaris segmentation, a small clew-like lesion corresponds to the above-mentioned tuft-shaped network. Moreover, in some cases, this glomerular lesion seems to be connected with the choroid through a small-caliber vessel [33].

OCT-A has confirmed the hypothesis that in most cases, the early appearance of type 3 neovascularization is characterized by an intraretinal vascular complex emerging from the DCP. This tuft-shaped intraretinal proliferation may be associated with evolving sub-RPE neovascular tissue, corresponding to a small clew-like lesion in the choriocapillaris segment. However, the presence of an early connection between the evolving sub-RPE neovascular tissue and the choroid does not allow for the exclusion, at least in some cases of type 3 neovascularization, of a possible choroidal origin.

Diabetic Retinopathy

Diabetic retinopathy (DR) is still considered the leading cause of blindness among the working-age population in industrially developed coun-

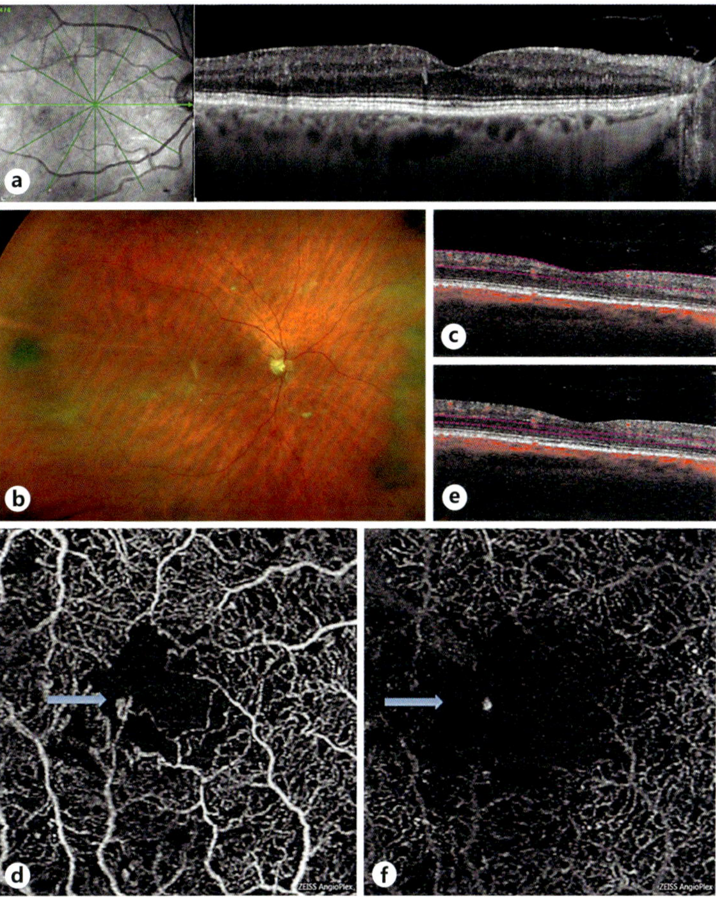

Fig. 3. A 68-year-old man with type 2 diabetes mellitus and poor glycemic control complained of floaters, secondary to vitreous hemorrhage. Best-corrected visual acuity in the right eye was 20/25, and fundus examination revealed proliferative diabetic retinopathy. **a** Enhanced depth imaging OCT disclosed the presence of an intraretinal hyperreflective lesion, without diabetic macular edema. **b** Panretinal fundus image showed multiple hemorrhages, microaneurysms, cotton wool spots and a residual vitreous hemorrhage. Structural B-scan (**c**) showed the level of SCP on OCT-A (**d**). **d** OCT-A scan (3 × 3 mm) of the SCP showed the presence of few microaneurysms, vessel dilatation, and perifoveal areas of nonperfusion, with rarefaction of the vascular network. A vascular abnormality (arrow) corresponding to an intraretinal microvascular abnormality is clearly visible on OCT-A (**d**), referring to the hyperreflective lesion seen on SD-OCT (**a**). B-scan (**e**) showed the level of DCP on OCT-A (**f**). **f** OCT-A scan (3 × 3 mm) of the DCP revealed a reduction of the vascularity, associated with enlargement of the FAZ, microaneurysms, focal capillary dilatation, and an hyperintense microvascular alteration (arrow).

tries [33]. There is evidence that a strict glycemic regimen and an effective blood pressure control can substantially reduce the risk of visual loss. However, diabetic macular edema (DME) and proliferative diabetic retinopathy (PDR) still remain the most sight-threatening complications. FA has been considered the gold standard for the analysis of the retinal vessels and capillary bed for at least 50 years. OCT with the more recent enhanced depth imaging technique is a noninvasive imaging tool, commonly used in the clinical daily routine, which provides accurate information of the retinal and choroidal morphology.

OCT-A is a new revolutionary method for the visualization of retinal and choroidal vasculature network that has rapidly reached a key role in the management of DR. OCT-A allows the evaluation of several alterations commonly present in DR, such as microaneurysms, DME, retinal ischemia and in some cases PDR [34–38]. Manual segmentation permits to identify vascular alterations and to correlate them with FA and OCT.

Enlargement of the Foveal Avascular Zone
Enlargement of the foveal avascular zone (FAZ) is frequently seen in patients with DR, due to an increased susceptibility to closure of the macular capillary bed. With OCT-A, the evaluation of the FAZ is easier than with conventional FA, due to the higher definition of the images. With the lay-

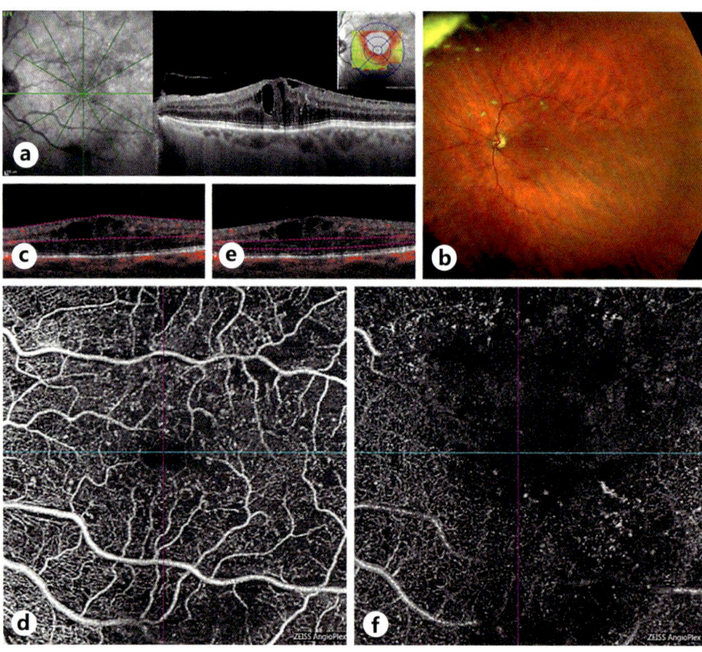

Fig. 4. Same patient as in Figure 1, suffering from PDR, complained significant metamorphopsia in the left eye (LE). Best-corrected visual acuity in LE was 20/50. **a** Enhanced depth imaging OCT revealed diabetic macular edema, located in the superior part of the macula, with large intraretinal cysts, hard exudates, and reduced choroidal thickness. **b** Panretinal fundus image showed multiple hemorrhages, microaneurysms, cotton wool spots, hard exudates, and preretinal hemorrhages. B-scan (**c**) showed the level of SCP on OCT-A (**d**). **d** OCT-A scan (6 × 6 mm) of the SCP showed the presence of multiple microaneurysms, vessel dilatation, and multiple areas of nonperfusion, with rarefaction of the vascular network. B-scan (**e**) showed the level of DCP on OCT-A (**f**). **f** OCT-A scan (6 × 6 mm) of the DCP revealed a large hyporeflective area due to the presence of diabetic macular area located in the superior part of the macula, multiple hyperintense vascular dilatation, and a reduction of the vascularity.

er-by-layer assessment of the retina and choroid, the presence of a network rarefaction is easy to show. Enlargement of the FAZ can affect both SCP and DCP in all stages of DR. However, enlargement of the FAZ and a lower vascular density are more frequently seen in patients with DME at the level of the DCP [36]. Diabetic macular ischemia is a serious complication of DR. With OCT-A, this dramatic condition is clearly appreciable without dye injection, showing a FAZ enlargement, capillary loss, and different degree of flow-void areas (Fig. 3–4).

Microaneurysms

Microvascular alteration of both SCP and DCP is frequently seen in patients with DME. Microaneurysms usually appear as focal hyperintense lesions with a roundish or fusiform aspect. Even if microaneurysms can be found in both SCP and DCP, more frequently they have been detected in the DCP, especially in patients with DME [37].

Diabetic Macular Edema

DME is conventionally characterized on biomicroscopy by retinal thickness and hard exudates. In patients with DME, OCT usually shows multiple intraretinal cystoid spaces and in some cases a serous retinal detachment, according to the degree of the disease. On OCT-A, the cystoid spaces inside the retina appear as hyporeflective, dark, roundish structures predominantly located in the inner nuclear-outer plexiform layer and the outer plexiform layer [35–38]. This hypointense aspect of the pseudocystic spaces is justified by the absence of blood flow.

Hard Exudates

Hard exudates in contrast are commonly seen as hyperintense areas in the neuroepithelial layer, using appropriate manual segmentation [38]. Hard exudates and microaneurysms have a similar focal hyperintense aspect on OCTA, and then they can, unfortunately, be confused [35]. How-

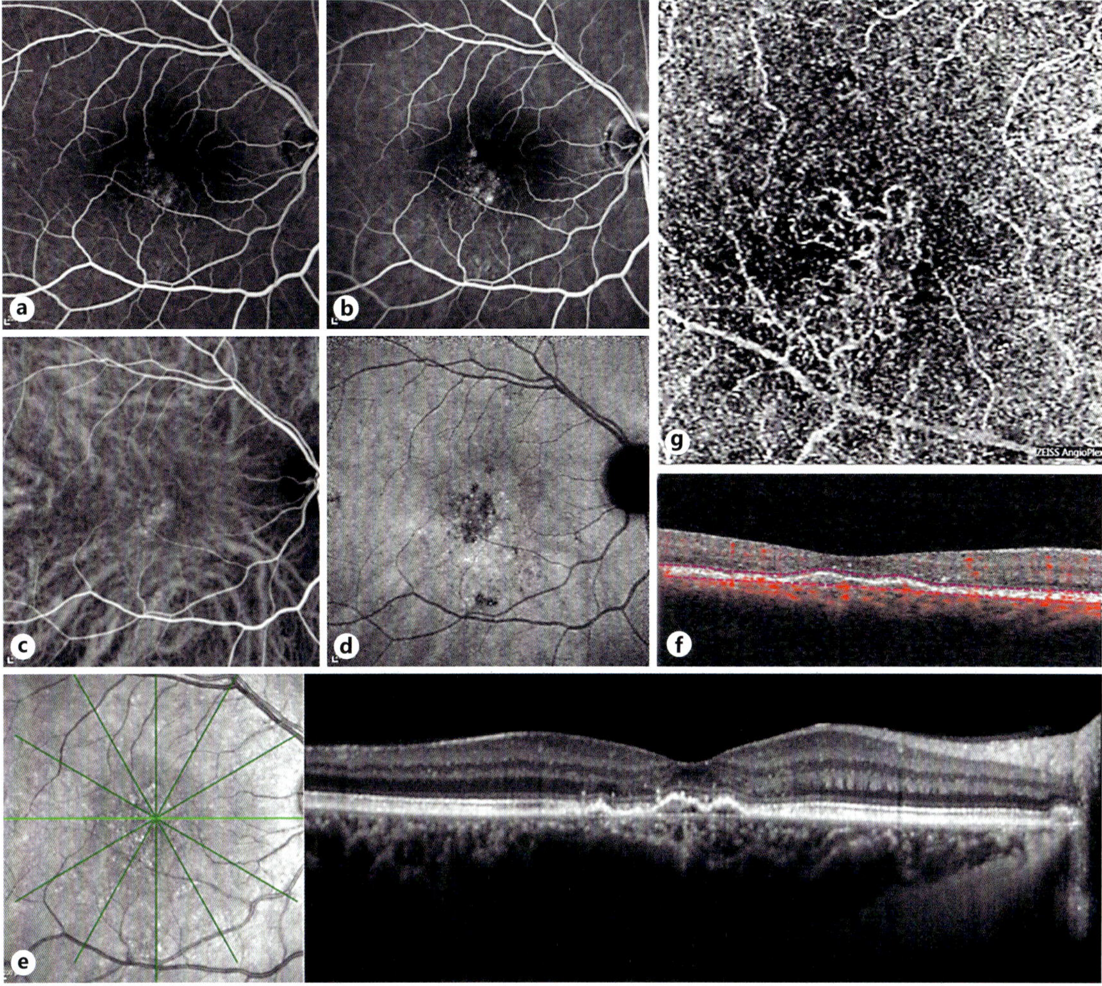

Fig. 5. A 48-year-old man suffering from chronic CSC in the right eye since 5 years complained of slight metamorphopsia with good visual acuity (best-corrected visual acuity 25/20). FA, early (**a**) and late (**b**) frames, and ICGA, early (**c**) and late (**d**) images showed inhomogeneous hyperfluorescence in the macular area. **e** Enhanced depth imaging OCT revealed the presence of a flat irregular PED, without subretinal fluid, dilation of choroidal vessels, and increased choroidal thickness. **f** B-scan showed the level of OCT-A. **g** OCT-A revealed the presence of clearly visible hyperreflective neovessels in the choriocapillaris.

ever, using a manual segmentation and correlating OCT-A with OCT or FA, these two entities can be easily differentiated.

Retinal Ischemia and Neovascularization
OCT-A, if appropriately addressed to the areas of retinal nonperfusion and neovascularization, can show significant vascular alterations. Using larger scans (such as 12 × 12 mm) and combining the different scans in a larger composite image, it is possible to obtain a clear visualization of the ischemic changes and preretinal vessels not only at the posterior pole but also at the midperiphery. This technique may be useful not only in the diagnosis but also in the monitoring of the treatment.

Choriocapillaris and Choroid Impairment

Choriocapillaris and choroid can be altered in diabetic patients. On OCT-A, a choriocapillary network rarefaction associated with areas of flow void can be detected in DR patients, secondary to the defects in vascular perfusion.

Pachychoroid Pigment Epitheliopathy

Central serous chorioretinopathy (CSC) is a common disease that primarily affects young or middle-aged men, characterized by subretinal fluid accumulation, often associated with RPE detachment [39]. It has been postulated that an abnormal choroidal hyperpermeability with vascular congestion is implicated in the pathogenesis of the disease, leading to an increased choroidal thickness and excessively dilated choroidal vessels [40]. Pachychoroid pigment epitheliopathy (PPE) has been considered a "forme fruste" of CSC, characterized by increased choroidal thickness, dilatation of the large outer choroidal vessels and RPE changes. According to this theory, the two entities share the same pathophysiology [41].

It has been theorized that patients with long-standing CSC and PPE may develop type 1 CNV, secondary to chronic RPE changes and serous PED. Type 1 CNV in PPE, which usually occurs overlying focal areas of choroidal thickening, has been called choroidal neovasculopathy [42, 43]

(Fig. 5). In addition, chronic CSC and PPE can worsen with the formation of polypoidal choroidal vasculopathy (PCV) [44].

However, the diagnosis of PCV is often challenging with FA and ICGA. Recently, the use of OCT-A allowed to detect with higher sensitivity and specificity than conventional imaging the presence of CNV in eyes with CSC [42]. Published studies showed that in chronic CSC and PPE, flat irregular PED may contain CNV. OCT-A revealed the presence of CNV more frequently than dye angiography, which consequently led to a change in the treatment option [45, 46].

ICGA has clearly shown that an impaired choroidal circulation is present in patients with CSC, characterized by multiple areas of choroidal vascular hyperpermeability. Based on this information, by using OCT-A, an increased choroidal vascular flow area has been detected in patients with CSC compared to healthy eyes [47]. The results of these studies confirmed the theory that the pathogenesis of CSC is related to a choroidal impairment.

Disclosure Statement

The authors declare that they have no conflicts of interest.

References

1 Stanga PE, Lim JI, Hamilton P: Indocyanine green angiography in chorioretinal diseases: indications and interpretation: an evidence-based update. Ophthalmology 2003;110:15–21; quiz 22–23.

2 Lopez-Saez MP, Ordoqui E, Tornero P, et al: Fluorescein-induced allergic reaction. Ann Allergy Asthma Immunol 1998;81:428–430.

3 Rabiolo A, Carnevali A, Bandello F, Querques G: Optical coherence tomography angiography: evolution or revolution? Exp Rev Ophthalmol 2016;11:243–245.

4 Huang D, Jia Y, Gao SS, Lumbroso B, Rispoli M: Optical coherence tomography angiography using the optovue device. Dev Ophthalmol 2016;56:6–12.

5 Kraus MF, Liu JJ, Schottenhamml J, et al: Quantitative 3D-OCT motion correction with tilt and illumination correction, robust similarity measure and regularization. Biomed Opt Express 2014;5: 2591–2613.

6 Kraus MF, Potsaid B, Mayer MA, et al: Motion correction in optical coherence tomography volumes on a per A-scan basis using orthogonal scan patterns. Biomed Opt Express 2012;3:1182–1199.

7 Rosenfeld PJ, Durbin MK, Roisman L, et al: ZEISS Angioplex™ spectral domain optical coherence tomography angiography: technical aspects. Dev Ophthalmol 2016;56:18–29.

8 Stanga PE, Tsamis E, Papayannis A, Stringa F, Cole T, Jalil A: Swept-source optical coherence tomography Angio™ (Topcon Corp, Japan): technology review. Dev Ophthalmol 2016;56:13–17.

9 Coscas G, Lupidi M, Coscas F: Heidelberg Spectralis optical coherence tomography angiography: technical aspects. Dev Ophthalmol 2016;56:1–5.

10 Pauleikhoff D, Spital G, Radermacher M, et al: A fluorescein and indocyanine green angiographic study of choriocapillaris in age-related macular disease. Arch Ophthalmol 1999;117:1353–1358.

11 Forte R, Querques G, Querques L, et al: Multimodal imaging of dry age-related macular degeneration. Acta Ophthalmol 2012;90:e281–e287.

12 Moult EM, Waheed NK, Novais EA, et al: Swept-source optical coherence tomography angiography reveals choriocapillaris alterations in eyes with nascent geographic atrophy and drusen-associated geographic atrophy. Retina 2016;36:S2–S11.

13 Coscas G, Lupidi M, Coscas F: Image analysis of optical coherence tomography angiography. Dev Ophthalmol 2016;56:30–36.

14 Querques G, Srour M, Massamba N, et al: Functional characterization and multimodal imaging of treatment-naive "quiescent" choroidal neovascularization. Invest Ophthalmol Vis Sci 2013;54:6886–6892.

15 Jia Y, Bailey ST, Wilson DJ, et al: Quantitative optical coherence tomography angiography of choroidal neovascularization in age-related macular degeneration. Ophthalmology 2014;121:1435–1444.

16 Gass JDM: Stereoscopic Atlas of Macular Diseases. Diagnosis and Treatment. St Louis, Mosby, 1997.

17 Carnevali A, Cicinelli MV, Capuano V, et al: Optical coherence tomography angiography: a useful tool for diagnosis of treatment-naïve quiescent choroidal neovascularization. Am J Ophthalmol 2016;169:189–198.

18 de Carlo TE, Bonini Filho MA, Chin AT, et al: Spectral-domain optical coherence tomography angiography of choroidal neovascularization. Ophthalmology 2015;122:1228–1238.

19 Iafea NA, Phasukkijwatanaa N, Sarraf D: Optical coherence tomography angiography of type 1 neovascularization in age-related macular degeneration. Dev Ophthalmol 2016;56:45–51.

20 Spaide RF, Klancnik JM Jr, Cooney MJ: Retinal vascular layers imaged by fluorescein angiography and optical coherence tomography angiography. JAMA Ophthalmol 2015;133:45–50.

21 Miere A, Semoun O, Cohen SY, et al: Optical coherence tomography angiography features of subretinal fibrosis in age-related macular. Retina 2015;35:2275–2284.

22 Kuehlewein L, Bansal M, Lenis TL, et al: Optical coherence tomography angiography of type 1 neovascularization in age-related macular degeneration. Am J Ophthalmol 2015;160:739–748.

23 Muakkassa NW, Chin AT, de Carlo T, et al: Characterizing the effect of anti-vascular endothelial growth factor therapy on treatment-naive choroidal neovascularization using optical coherence tomography angiography. Retina 2015;35:2252–2259.

24 Moult E, Choi W, Waheed NK, et al: Ultrahigh-speed sweptsource OCT angiography in exudative AMD. Ophthalmic Surg Lasers Imaging Retina 2014;45:496–505.

25 Cohen SY, Creuzot-Garcher C, Darmon J, et al: Types of choroidal neovascularization in newly diagnosed exudative age-related macular degeneration. Br J Ophthalmol 2007;91:1173–1176.

26 Lopez PF, Lambert HM, Grossniklaus HE, et al: Well-defined subfoveal choroidal neovascular membranes in age-related macular degeneration. Ophthalmology 1993;100:415–422.

27 El Ameen A, Cohen SY, Semoun O, et al: Type 2 neovascularization secondary to age-related macular degeneration imaged by optical coherence tomography angiography. Retina 2015;35:2212–2218.

28 Spaide RF, Fujimoto JG, Waheed NK: Image artifacts in optical coherence tomography angiography. Retina 2015;35:2163–2180.

29 Freund KB, Ho IV, Barbazetto IA, et al: Type 3 neovascularization: the expanded spectrum of retinal angiomatous proliferation. Retina 2008;28:201–211.

30 Yannuzzi LA, Negrao S, Iida T, et al: Retinal angiomatous proliferation in age-related macular degeneration. Retina 2001;21:416–434.

31 Gass JD, Agarwal A, Lavina AM, et al: Focal inner retinal hemorrhages in patients with drusen: an early sign of occult choroidal neovascularization and chorioretinal anastomosis. Retina 2003;23:741–751.

32 Yannuzzi LA, Freund KB, Takahashi BS: Review of retinal angiomatous proliferation or type 3 neovascularization. Retina 2008;28:375–384.

33 Miere A, Querques G, Semoun O, et al: Optical coherence tomography angiography in early type 3 neovascularization. Retina 2015;35:2236–2241.

34 Klein R, Klein BE, Moss SE, Davis MD, DeMets DL: The Wisconsin epidemiologic study of diabetic retinopathy. III. Prevalence and risk of diabetic retinopathy when age at diagnosis is 30 or more years. Arch Ophthalmol 1984;102:527–532.

35 Coscas G, Lupidi M, Coscas F: Optical coherence tomography in diabetic maculopathy; in Bandello F, Zarbin MA, Lattanzio R, Zucchiatti I (eds): Management of Diabetic Retinopathy. Dev Ophthalmol. Basel, Karger, 2017, vol 60, pp 38–49.

36 Lee J, Moon BG, Cho AR, Yoon YH: Optical coherence tomography angiography of DME and its association with anti-VEGF treatment response. Ophthalmology 2016;123:2368–2375.

37 Hasegawa N, Nozaki M, Takase N, Yoshida M, Ogura Y: New insights into microaneurysms in the deep capillary plexus detected by optical coherence tomography angiography in diabetic macular edema. Invest Ophthalmol Vis Sci 2016;57:348–355.

38 Stanga PE, Papayannis A, Tsamis E, et al: New findings in diabetic maculopathy and proliferative disease by swept-source optical coherence tomography angiography; in Bandello F, Souied EH, Querques G (eds): OCT Angiography in Retinal and Macular Diseases. Dev Ophthalmol. Basel, Karger, 2016, vol 56, pp 113–121.

39 Gass JD: Pathogenesis of disciform detachment of the neuroepithelium. Am J Ophthalmol 1967;63:1–139.

40 Imamura Y, Fujiwara T, Margolis R, Spaide RF: Enhanced depth imaging coherence tomography of the choroid in central serous chorioretinopathy. Retina 2009;29:1469–1473.

41 Warrow DJ, Hoang QV, Freund KB: Pachychoroid pigment epitheliopathy. Retina 2013;33:1659–1672.

42 Bonini Filho MA, de Carlo TE, Ferrara D, et al: Association of choroidal neovascularization and central serous chorioretinopathy with optical coherence tomography angiography. JAMA Ophthalmol 2015;133:899–906.

43 Pang CE, Freund KB: Pachychoroid neovasculopathy. Retina 2015;35:1–9.

44 Ahuja RM, Downes SM, Stanga PE, Koh
AH, Vingerling JR, Bird AC: Polypoidal
choroidal vasculopathy and central serous chorioretinopathy. Ophthalmology
2001;108:1009–1010.

45 Bousquet E, Bonnin S, Mrejen S, Krivo-
sic V, Tadayoni R, Gaudric A: Optical
coherence tomography angiography of
flat irregular pigment epithelium detachment in chronic central serous chorioretinopathy. Retina DOI: 10.1097/
IAE.0000000000001580.

46 Azar G, Wolff B, Mauget-Faÿsse M,
Rispoli M, Savastano MC, Lumbroso B:
Pachychoroid neovasculopathy: aspect
on optical coherence tomography angiography. Acta Ophthalmol 2017;95:421–
427.

47 Nicolò M, Rosa R, Musetti D, Musolino
M, Saccheggiani M, Traverso CE: Choroidal vascular flow area in central serous chorioretinopathy using swept-
source optical coherence tomography
angiography. Invest Ophthalmol Vis Sci
2017;58:2002–2010.

Prof. Giuseppe Querques
Department of Ophthalmology
University Vita-Salute, IRCCS Ospedale San Raffaele
Via Olgettina 60, IT–20132 Milan (Italy)
E-Mail giuseppe.querques@hotmail.it

Querques · Sacconi · Carnevali · Querques · Zucchiatti · Bandello

Cunha-Vaz J, Koh A (eds): Imaging Techniques.
ESASO Course Series. Basel, Karger, 2018, vol 10, pp 65–87 (DOI: 10.1159/000487413)

Autofluorescence Imaging

Maximilian Pfau · Monika Fleckenstein · Steffen Schmitz-Valckenberg · Frank G. Holz

Department of Ophthalmology, University of Bonn, Bonn, Germany

Abstract

Fundus autofluorescence allows for spatially resolved mapping of physiological and pathological fluorophores of the ocular fundus. The dominant retinal autofluorescence intensity using a blue excitation light arises from lipofuscin (LF) within the lysosomal compartment of postmitotic retinal pigment epithelium (RPE) cells. LF accumulation, originating from incomplete degradation of photoreceptor outer segment disks, represents a hallmark of RPE cell ageing. Excessive accumulation of LF granules in the lysosomal compartment of RPE cells signifies a downstream pathogenic pathway in several hereditary and complex retinal diseases.

Technical Background

Fundus Autofluorescence

Fundus autofluorescence (FAF) imaging is a non-invasive imaging method for in vivo mapping of naturally or pathologically occurring fluorophores of the ocular fundus (Fig. 1). The dominant sources of the FAF signal using a blue excitation light are fluorophores amassing in lipofuscin (LF) granules in postmitotic retinal pigment epithelium (RPE) cells [1]. In the absence of RPE cells, various minor fluorophores including elastin and collagen, e.g. in choroidal blood vessel walls, may also become visible [2]. The RPE comprises a polygonal monolayer between the neurosensory retina and the choroid [3]. LF accumulation – originating from incomplete degradation of photoreceptor outer segment disks – represents a hallmark of RPE cell ageing [3–6]. Multiple lines of evidence indicate that adverse effects of LF accumulation constitute a common downstream pathogenic mechanism in various monogenic macular and retinal dystrophies as well as multifactorial complex retinal diseases such as age-related macular degeneration (AMD) [6, 7]. Seemingly, once formed, the RPE cell does not

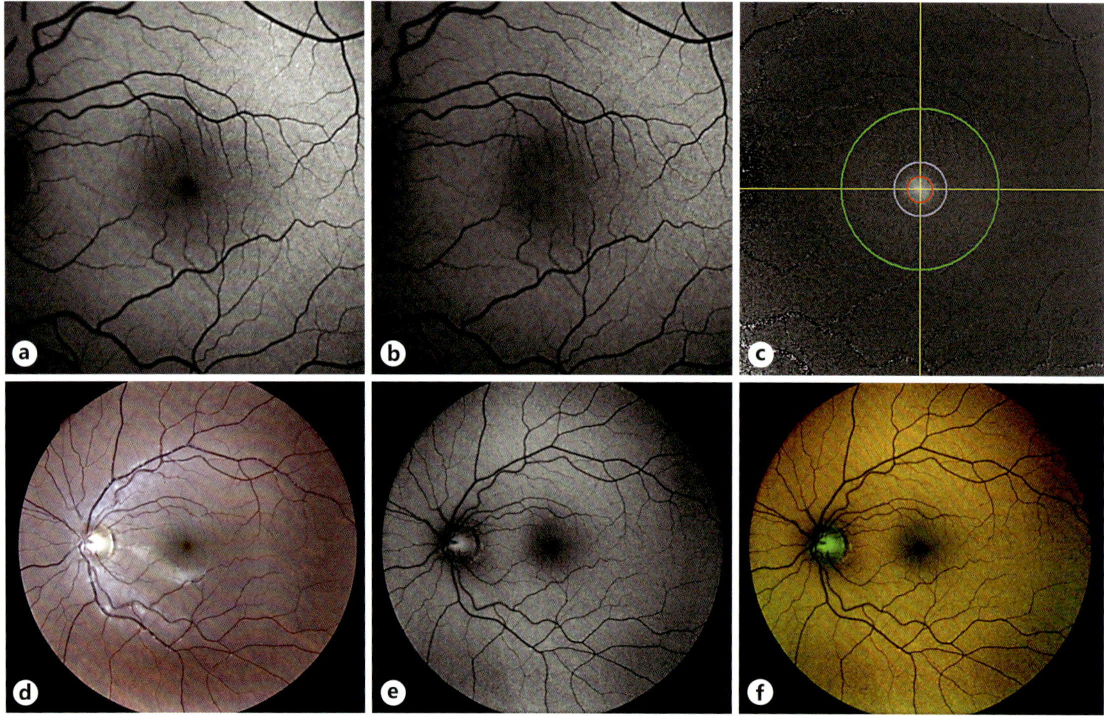

Fig. 1. a, **b** Blue-light (BAF, excitation 488 nm) and green-light fundus autofluorescence (GAF, excitation 518 nm) images of a healthy subject. Notably, the BAF image centrally shows a decreased intensity due to the macular pigment (lutein, zeaxanthin, and meso-zeaxanthin) absorbing the short-wavelength excitation light. **c** Measurement of the macular pigment optical density based on the BAF and GAF images. **d** A wide-field color fundus photography. Corresponding BAF (**e**) and emission-color-resolved BAF (**f**). Notably, structures rich in collagen (i.e., lamina cribrosa of the optic disc) exhibit a rather greenish autofluorescence, while the retinal pigment epithelium exhibits a more yellowish autofluorescence.

have any means of either degrading or transporting LF granules to the extracellular space through exocytosis [8–12].

Rhodopsin and "Bleaching"

Rhodopsin, the visual pigment of rod photoreceptors has a major influence on FAF images. With an absorption spectrum peak at 498 nm, it absorbs the excitation light [13]. However, under continued exposure to the blue excitation light, rhodopsin undergoes photoisomerization losing its absorptive properties. This results in an increase in the FAF signal of up to 30% termed "bleaching" [14]. In a clinical setting, bleaching is typically visible if a wide-field image (i.e., 55°) is taken immediately after an initial 30° image (Fig. 2) [14]. In retinal dystrophies with photoreceptor dysfunction such as cone-rod dystrophy, Stargardt disease and choroidermia, "bleaching" is less apparent [14].

Green-Light Autofluorescence and Macular Pigment

Various functions have been suggested for macular pigment, including filtration of blue light reducing photodamage and glare, minimization of the effects of chromatic aberration on visual acuity, improvement in fine-detail discrimination, and enhancement of contrast sensitivity [15–17]. While the interindividual variability of the con-

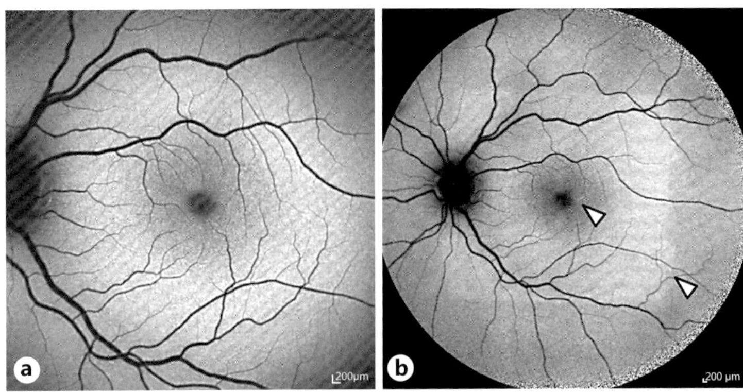

Fig. 2. A 30° fundus autofluorescence (FAF) image (**a**) and a 55° FAF image (**b**) taken immediately after the first image. An increase in the FAF signal termed "bleaching" is clearly visible as indicated by the arrowheads. Further, the fixation target (blue cross) may also result in bleaching.

centration of macular pigment is high, its spatial distribution is relatively uniform across individuals. It shows a peak concentration at the foveal center and decreases significantly with eccentricity, with negligible concentrations at about 8° of eccentricity [15–17]. Thus, measuring the intensity of FAF simultaneously with two wavelengths, one well absorbed and the other minimally absorbed by macular pigment, provides a measurement of the macular pigment optical density (MPOD) [18]. Evaluation of the fovea with blue-light autofluorescence (BAF, excitation 488 nm) imaging may be challenging, since macular pigment (lutein, zeaxanthin, and meso-zeaxanthin) absorbs the short-wavelength excitation light (Fig. 1) [18, 19]. In contrast to BAF imaging, green-light autofluorescence (GAF, excitation 518 nm) imaging is not significantly affected by macular pigment due to a lack of absorption [18]. Thus, GAF imaging allows for even more precise assessment of small, central changes including the differentiation between foveal atrophy and foveal sparing in geographic atrophy (GA) secondary to AMD (Fig. 3) [19, 20].

Near-Infrared Autofluorescence
The use of excitation and emission wavelengths in the red end of the spectrum for near-infrared autofluorescence (NIR-AF) imaging allows for mapping of the topographic distribution of fluorophores other than LF [21–23]. Gibbs et al. [24]

postulated that melanosomes in the RPE and choroid are the likely predominant source of the NIR-AF signal. Schmitz-Valckenberg et al. [25] examined the distribution of this NIR-AF signal in retinal cross-sections of a human donor eye. Correlating these ex vivo autofluorescence measurements to in vivo findings in a rat animal model, the authors also concluded that the NIR-AF signal was spatially confined to the RPE monolayer and melanin within the choroid [25]. NIR-AF imaging may be easily performed in vivo using the indocyanine green angiography mode of a scanning laser ophthalmoscope, i.e. without dye injection [21–23].

Acquisition of Autofluorescence Imaging
Multiple devices may be used for noninvasive, in vivo recoding of autofluorescence images. The pioneering fundus spectrophotometer by Delori et al. [1] allowed for confocal multichannel spectral analysis of emission spectra (500–800 nm) with seven excitation wavelengths (430 and 550 nm) of small retinal areas (2° visual angle). In a hallmark study, Delori et al. [1] were able to demonstrate that the autofluorescence emission form the fundus is broad, ranging from 500 to 800 nm. The intensity increases with age [1]. The peak emission at 620–630 nm (optimal excitation at 510 nm) was in line with the assumption that LF constitutes the dominant fluorophore [1].

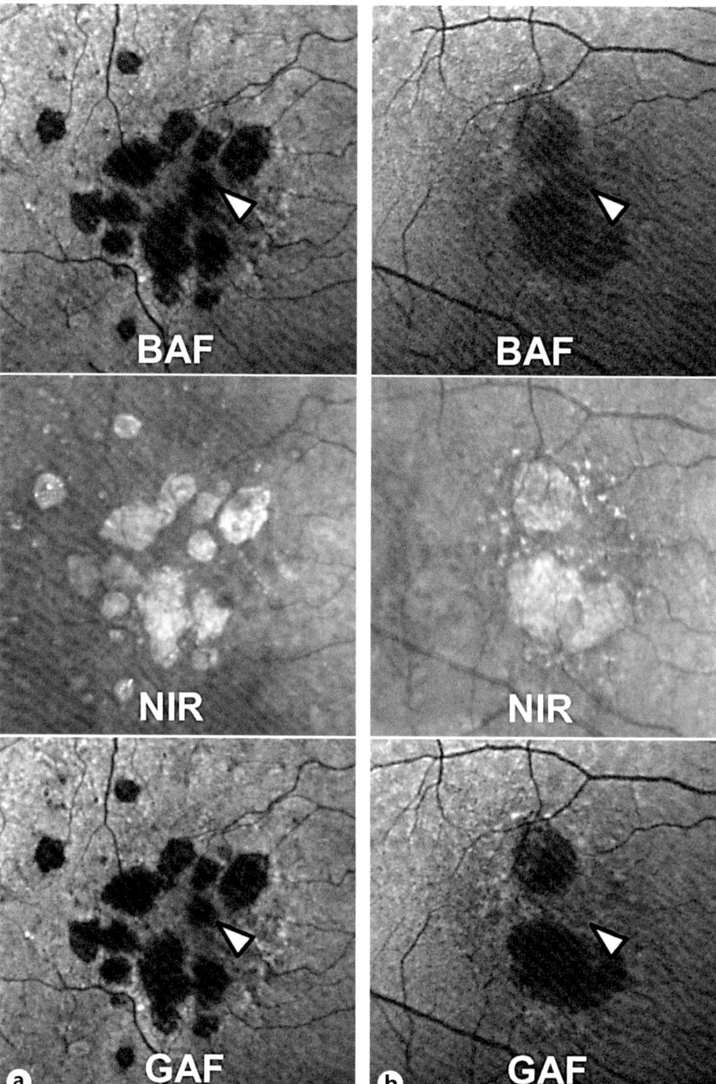

Fig. 3. Blue-light autofluorescence (BAF, excitation 488 nm), near-infrared reflectance (NIR), and green-light autofluorescence (GAF, excitation 518 nm) of 2 exemplary patients (**a** and **b**, respectively) with geographic atrophy secondary to age-related macular degeneration are shown. As indicated by the arrowheads, it is difficult to assess on the BAF image whether the fovea is atrophic or spared. The NIR and GAF images confirm the presence of atrophy. In patient B, the NIR and GAF image confirm that the fovea is spared.

While fundus camera-based FAF imaging is convenient given that most cameras designed for fluorescein angiography may be used, it exhibits several disadvantages [26]. Absorption and scattering of the crystalline lens as well as scattered light due to the nonconfocality limit the image quality [26]. Delori et al. [26] described a modified fundus camera for FAF imaging to reduce the scattering and fluorescence from the crystalline lens by inserting an aperture in the illumination optics of the camera. The resulting field of view (diameter of 13°), however, limited the applicability [26]. Spaide [27] described another modification of a commercially available fundus camera to reduce the effects of the crystalline lens. He suggested shifting the excitation wavelength towards the green spectrum and the emission wavelength towards the yellow-orange spectrum with relatively inexpensive additional filters [27].

The resolution of FAF could be greatly enhanced by confocal scanning laser ophthalmoscopy (cSLO) imaging [28]. cSLO optimally addresses the limitations of fundus camera-based FAF imaging. These are interference of the crystalline lens and the low intensity of the retinal signal [28, 29]. In cSLO FAF imaging, the laser is swept across the fundus in a raster pattern and the emitted light at each point is registered after passing through a confocal pinhole suppressing fluorescence from the crystalline lens [28, 29]. It was first applied by von Rückmann et al. [29] in a clinical setting. The cSLO system for FAF imaging by Heidelberg Engineering (formerly Heidelberg retina angiograph, now Heidelberg Spectralis [Heidelberg Engineering, Heidelberg, Germany]) is currently the most widely used system. A key advantage of the Heidelberg Spectralis system is the possibility of simultaneous spectral-domain optical coherence tomography (SD-OCT) and cSLO FAF imaging. This allows for precise correlation of FAF findings with SD-OCT data. Other systems, including the Rodenstock cSLO and the Zeiss (Carl Zeiss Meditec, Oberkochen, Germany) prototype SM for FAF imaging, are no longer commercially available. More recently, the F-10 cSLO platform (Nidek, Gamagori, Japan) and the Eidon AF SLO system (CenterVue, Padova, Italy) have been introduced.

Wide-field imaging allows for imaging of even larger retinal areas as compared to typical cSLO FAF imaging with a field of 30° × 30°. An additional lens for the Heidelberg cSLO extends the field to 55°. Alternatively, montage images can be (semi-)automatically generated with most FAF fundus cameras and FAF cSLO platforms with alignment of individual frames. The wide-field scanning laser ophthalmoscope P200Tx (Optos) allows for FAF SLO acquisition in less than 2 s using a green light excitation (532 nm) [30–33]. Similarly, the CLARUS 500 (Zeiss) allows for wide-field acquisition of BAF (435–500 nm) and GAF (500–585 nm) images with a field of view of 200°. These techniques allow for longitudinal assessment of diseases affecting the peripheral retina beyond the vascular arcades.

In a research setting, quantitative autofluorescence (qAF) imaging has been introduced allowing for reliable measurement and comparison of FAF intensities [34, 35]. Briefly, the Heidelberg qAF cSLO incorporates a stable standard fluorescent reference [34, 35]. Thus, differences of the laser power and detector gain across multiple sites, which affect the FAF intensity, can be accounted for in order to determine qAF values [34, 35]. Further, age and axial length are also accounted for. Thus, qAF values reflect FAF intensities relative to those which would be measured in an emmetropic eye with average ocular dimensions [34, 35].

Another novel imaging instrument for research purposes is fluorescence lifetime imaging ophthalmoscopy (FLIO). Schweitzer et al. [36–38] were the first to perform FLIO in vivo. Hereby, the lifetime of the fluorophore signal, rather than its intensity is quantified [36–38]. The fluorescence lifetime is an intrinsic property of a fluorophore, but may be affected by external factors, such as temperature, polarity, and the presence of fluorescence quenchers. FLIO allows therefore for the mapping of metabolic processes in vivo [2]. Generally, organic fluorophores decay within several nanoseconds [2].

Complex Diseases

Age-Related Macular Degeneration
Intermediate AMD
Drusen, the hallmark finding of intermediate AMD, represent a variety of extracellular deposits between the basal lamina of the RPE and the inner layer of Bruch's membrane [39]. These include soft drusen (small [diameter ≤63 μm], medium [64–124 μm], large [≥125 μm]), hard drusen, cuticular drusen, and crystalline drusen [39]. Generally, larger drusen are more frequently associated with FAF abnormalities compared to smaller

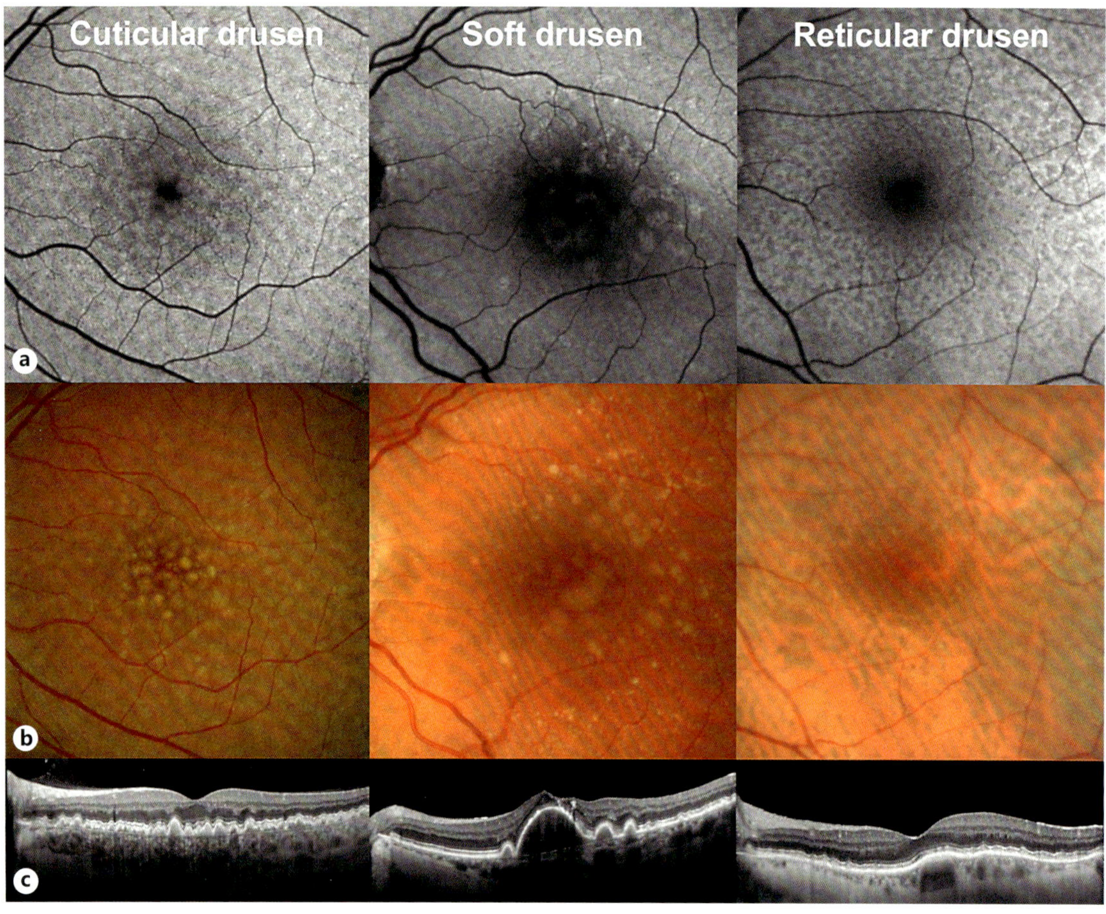

Fig. 4. Fundus autofluorescence (FAF) images (**a**), color fundus photographs (CFP; **b**), and foveal horizontal spectral-domain optical coherence tomography (SD-OCT; **c**) scans of 3 patients. Cuticular drusen are characterized by a fine granular pattern of increased FAF signal and a saw-tooth pattern on SD-OCT. Soft drusen exhibit patchy increased FAF. Reticular drusen may be more easily detected on FAF images compared to CFP images. The dot- and ribbon-like pattern corresponds to spike-like lesion on the SD-OCT.

drusen (Fig. 4) [40]. Large drusen exhibit most commonly increased autofluorescence but may also exhibit normal or decreased autofluorescence (Fig. 4) [40]. Cuticular drusen (also known as basal laminar drusen) – an early-onset-drusen phenotype that shows a pattern of uniform small (25–75 μm), slightly raised, yellow subretinal nodules – are an exception [41]. Cuticular drusen are clearly notable on FAF images despite their small size, but are most easily recognized on fluorescein angiography imaging exhibiting the typi-

cal "stars-in-the-sky" pattern [41]. The various phenotypic differences of drusen in FAF imaging presumably reflect the differential molecular composition of the accumulated extracellular material. Further, so-called reticular drusen (also known as reticular pseudodrusen and subretinal drusenoid deposits) have been described in the setting of AMD (Fig. 4) [40, 42–44]. These were shown to be highly prevalent in eyes with late AMD and associated with a high risk of progression to late-stage AMD [45–48]. On FAF images,

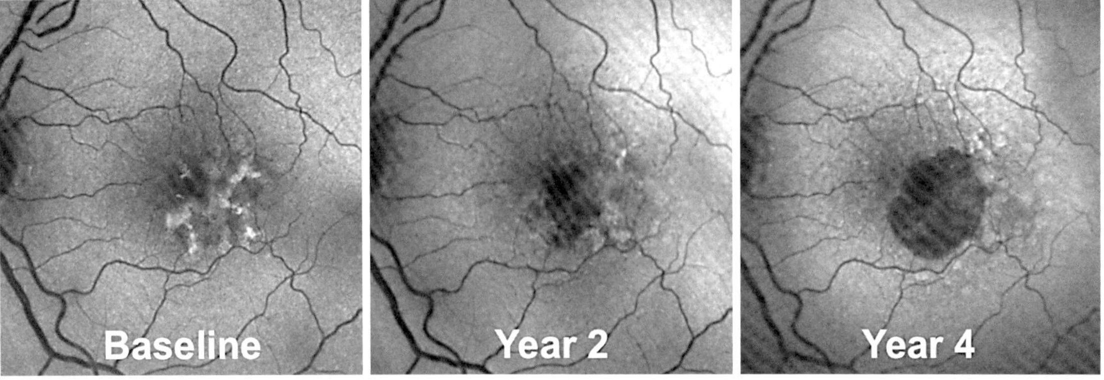

Fig. 5. Serial fundus autofluorescence (FAF) images of a patient showing a long-term course of age-related macular degeneration. At the first visit, the patient presented with an avascular pigment epithelium detachment (PED) characterized by a cartwheel-like FAF pattern. The flattening of the PED resulted in geographic atrophy hallmarked by the well-demarcated definitely decreased FAF signal.

reticular drusen are visible either as a network of broad, interlacing ribbons or as dot-like lesions exhibiting decreased autofluorescence and may be classified accordingly [49]. Besides drusen, focal hypo- and hyperpigmentation represent the other hallmark finding in intermediate AMD [39]. Focal hyperpigmentation has been attributed to localized areas of RPE cell hypertrophy and anterior migration that may be associated with clumps of pigmented cells in the sub-RPE or subretinal space. Hyperpigmentary lesions show typically increased autofluorescence on FAF images [40]. The FAF classification for intermediate AMD based on the natural history Fundus Autofluorescence in AMD (FAM) study, was shown to predict visual loss [40, 50]. Especially the patchy FAF pattern was shown to be prognostic for future severe visual loss [51]. In a different cohort, the patchy FAF pattern was also shown to be the most frequent pattern in eyes with subsequent CNV development [50]. The identification and systematic comparison of risk factors in intermediate AMD for the development late AMD still constitutes a subject of intense research as evidenced by the ongoing EU-funded MACUSTAR project and the AMD Ryan Initiative Study (ARIS).

Recently, Gliem et al. [52] demonstrated using qAF that the qAF levels in patients with early and intermediate AMD are rather low compared to age-matched controls. Thus, despite localized lesions with increased autofluorescence, the overall LF levels in the RPE might be rather subnormal in eyes with AMD [52]. In terms of fluorescence lifetime, eyes with AMD were shown to exhibit overall elongated mean lifetimes using FLIO [53]. Localized long fluorescence lifetimes were shown to correspond to intraretinal hyperreflective foci as seen on SD-OCT [53]. Localized short fluorescence lifetimes were occasionally also observed and co-localized with deposits in the area of the outer photoreceptor segments [53].

Geographic Atrophy
In GA, the nonexudative late-stage manifestation of AMD, FAF imaging has been validated as both a clinical endpoint and a prognostic biomarker. The loss of RPE and its inherent fluorophores in GA correlates with well-defined areas of decreased autofluorescence [54, 55], allowing for precise manual, semiautomatic, or automatic GA segmentation methods based on FAF imaging (Fig. 5) [56–62]. Hereby, the semiautomatic region-growing image analysis approach has been

integrated in the RegionFinder™ software (Heidelberg Engineering) [58–60]. Schmitz-Valckenberg et al. [59] demonstrated that the software allows for reproducible delineation of atrophy with high interrater agreement. A new update, first described by Lindner et al. [60], allows for combined grading of FAF and near-infrared reflectance cSLO images to differentiate between foveal atrophy and foveal sparing. In eyes with foveal-sparing GA, Lindner et al. [60] were able to demonstrate that centrifugal progression is significantly faster than centripetal progression. While the underlying pathomechanism for differential GA progression remains unknown, local factors may be operative that appear to protect the foveal retina [60].

The RegionFinder™ software is used to quantify the primary outcome measure in (ongoing) clinical trials (NCT02247531, NCT02247479, NCT02087085, http://clinicaltrials.gov). In this context, FAF imaging has been recommended among other imaging modalities for the detection and measurement of atrophy by the CAM group (Classification of Atrophy Meeting) [63]. Recently, Pfau et al. [20] demonstrated that green-light FAF imaging provides even better interrater agreement, suggesting that its use may be preferable in clinical trials examining the change in lesion size as a clinical endpoint (Fig. 3). It must be noted, that very early atrophic lesions in the absence of drusen (nascent geographic atrophy) may be characterized by both increased and decreased autofluorescence impeding the quantification of these small lesions [64].

In terms of prognosis, it was shown in the multicenter longitudinal natural history FAM study that the area of increased autofluorescence surrounding GA is strongly correlated with disease progression [65]. Moreover, Holz et al. [57] could identify nine different FAF subphenotypes based on the presence and shape of perilesional increased autofluorescence: none, focal, diffuse (reticular, branching, trickling, fine granular, fine granular with peripheral punctate spots), banded, and patchy (Fig. 6). The prognostic value of this classification for the upcoming progression rates was validated in other cohorts [66–68]. Two of the FAF phenotypes were shown to differ genetically from the other phenotypes. The "fine granular with peripheral punctate spots" phenotype was shown to be associated with *ABCA4* mutations and is therefore now classified as late-onset Stargardt disease (Fig. 6) [69]. Patients exhibiting the diffuse-trickling GA phenotype (characterized by lobular atrophy with "grayish" signal within areas of GA) were also shown to exhibit a remarkably different genetic risk profile from patients with other GA phenotypes (Fig. 6) [70]. However, no disease-specific mutations could be identified yet [70]. Interestingly, patients with diffuse-trickling GA exhibit higher progression rates, more pronounced choroidal thinning and a higher rate of cardiovascular comorbidity as compared to patients with other GA phenotypes [71].

Neovascular AMD

Early type 1 (occult) choroidal neovascularization may not be readily detectable on FAF images due to the intact RPE [72, 73]. In contrast, type 2 classic neovascularization lesion may show decreased autofluorescence due to the blockage of the RPE signal by the fibrovascular subretinal lesion [72, 73]. Nearly 40% of treatment-naive eyes exhibit a ring or streaks of increased autofluorescence associated with (former) subretinal fluid and disruption of the ellipsoid zone in SD-OCT [74]. Hereby, the increased autofluorescence may most likely be explained by the loss of photoreceptor outer segments (including the rhodopsin) resulting in a window defect (cf. "bleaching") [74]. Heimes et al. [75] analyzed the predictive value FAF imaging in 95 eyes undergoing intravitreal anti-VEGF therapy. A significantly worse outcome in visual acuity was observed for eyes with an increased autofluorescence signal within the central 500 μm [75].

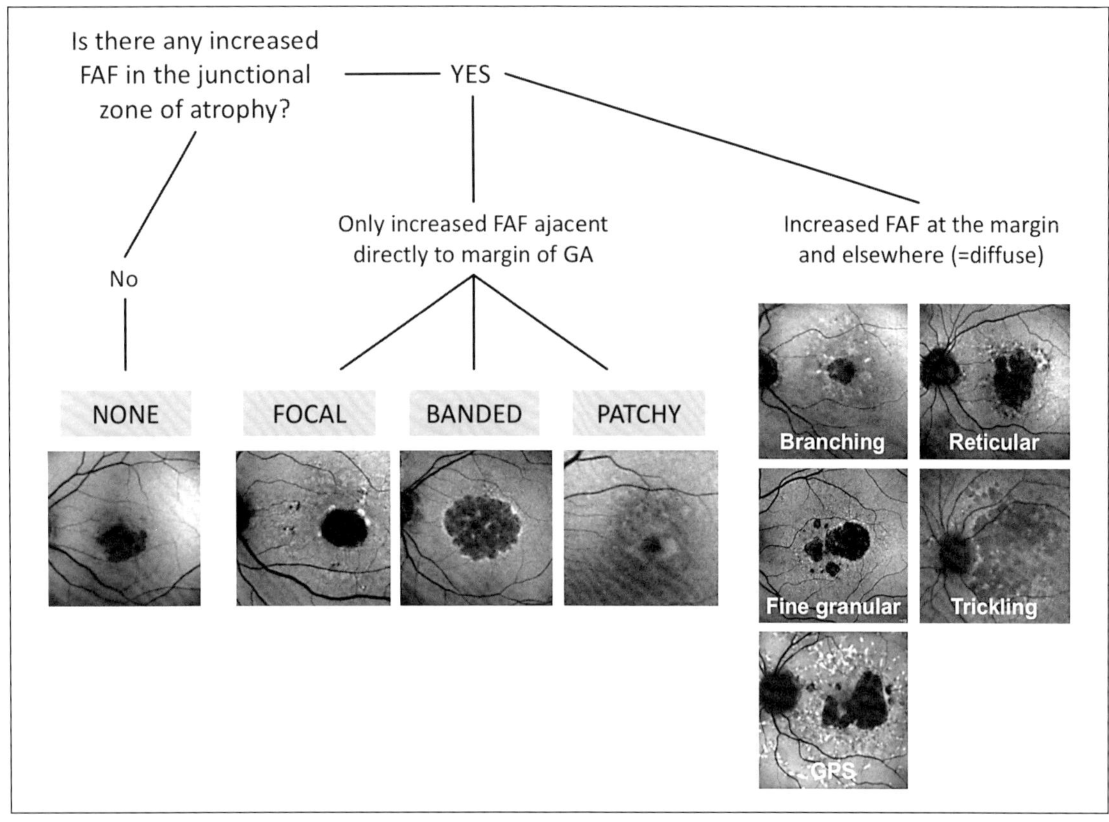

Fig. 6. Geographic atrophy (GA) secondary to age-related macular degeneration may be classified according to the junctional fundus autofluorescence (FAF) signal. Four of these patterns are characterized by no increased FAF signal or increased FAF signal only directly in continuity with the GA lesion. The five diffuse patterns present with increased FAF signal elsewhere. The diffuse-trickling pattern exhibits the most rapid progression rates and appears to be associated cardiovascular comorbidity. The "fine granular with peripheral punctate spots" (GPS) phenotype was shown to be associated with *ABCA4* mutations and is therefore now classified as late-onset Stargardt disease.

Retinal Pigment Epithelial Tears

Vascularized pigment epithelial detachment, a subtype of neovascular AMD, may be complicated spontaneously or following photodynamic therapy or anti-VEGF therapy by tears of the RPE (RIP) [76]. On FAF imaging, RIP is characterized by well-demarcated decreased autofluorescence due to the absence of RPE, with an adjacent region of increased autofluorescence corresponding to the retracted RPE (Fig. 7) [76–78]. Interestingly, reappearance of the fluorescence within the area of the RIP has been observed, which might potentially represent "RPE resurfacing" (Fig. 7) [76, 78, 79].

Diabetic Retinopathy

Diabetic retinopathy, the second most common retinal cause of blindness, may show a variety of abnormalities on FAF imaging [80]. Dot and blot hemorrhages and hard exudates exhibit typically decreased autofluorescence and may be differentiated based on shape. Cystoid macular edema is typically visible as a petaloid pattern of increased autofluorescence (Fig. 8) [80]. This has been attributed to the displacement of luteal pigment, since cysts are mostly located in the outer plexiform and inner nuclear layer [80]. Indeed, Bessho et al. [81] reported that increased

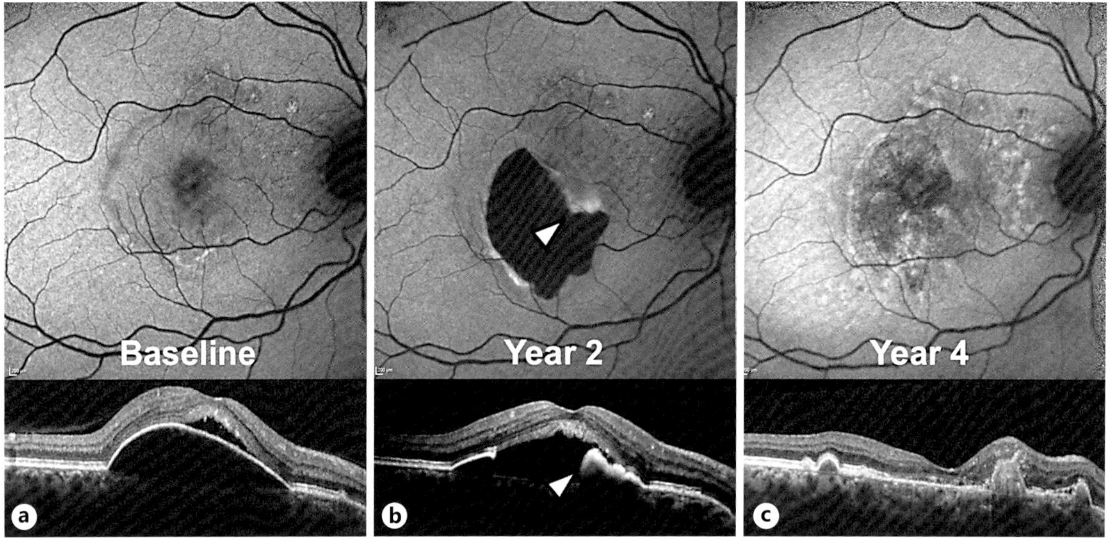

Fig. 7. a Long-term course of a tear of the retinal pigment epithelium (RIP) on fundus autofluorescence and spectral-domain optical coherence tomography. The RIP is visible as a well-demarcated area of decreased autofluorescence due to absence of retinal pigment epithelium, with adjacent focally increased autofluorescence corresponding to the retracted retinal pigment epithelium (arrowheads in **b**). **c** Interestingly, reappearance of the fluorescence within the area of the RIP is observable.

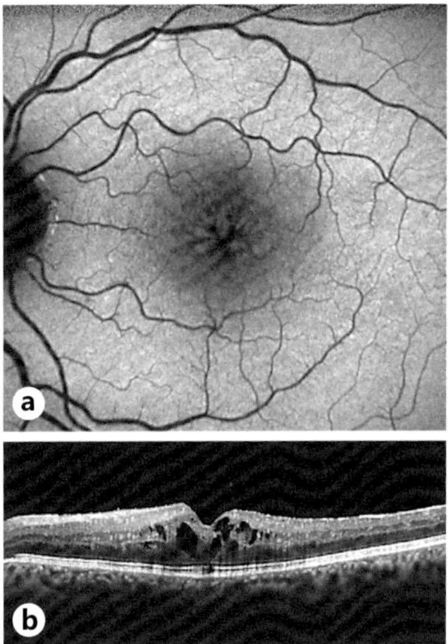

Fig. 8. Fundus autofluorescence (FAF; **a**) and spectral-domain optical coherence tomography (**b**) show diabetic macular edema. Cystoid macular edema is typically visible as increased FAF, which is attributable to the displacement of luteal pigment, since cysts are mostly located in the outer plexiform and inner nuclear layer.

autofluorescence due to cystoid macular edema was always observed on FAF imaging with an excitation wavelength of 488 nm, while it was rarely observed on FAF imaging with an excitation wavelength of 580 nm, demonstrating that the increased autofluorescence in cystoid macular edema represents "relatively" increased autofluorescence, due to lateral displacement of luteal pigments.

Central Serous Chorioretinopathy
Serous retinal detachment, the hallmark feature of central serous chorioretinopathy, results in areas with decreased autofluorescence due to the blockage of signal by subretinal fluid [82]. Some patients also show granular and punctuate increased autofluorescence that typically corresponds to subretinal precipitates at the level of photoreceptor outer segments on SD-OCT (Fig. 9) [82]. In chronic cases lasting longer than 6 months, 85% of patients were shown to exhibit

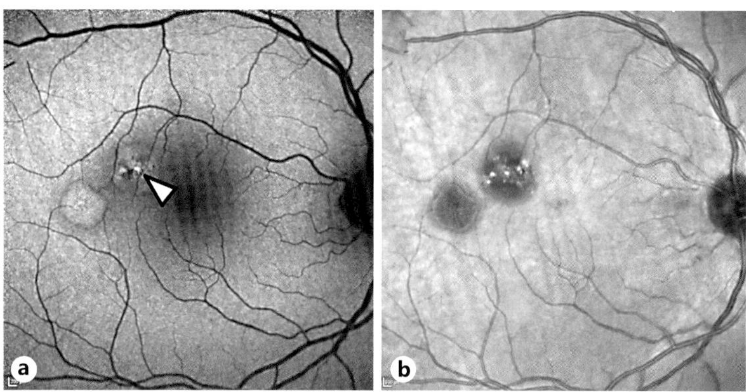

Fig. 9. Fundus autofluorescence (FAF; **a**) and near-infrared reflectance (**b**) show two small serous retinal detachments, the hallmark feature of central serous chorioretinopathy. Subretinal fluid may result in blockage of the FAF signal but also in increased FAF signal if the photoreceptor outer segments are missing (reduction of rhodopsin, c.f. "bleaching"). Spots with increased FAF (arrowhead) typically correlated with hyperreflective clumps in the regions of the photoreceptor outer segments on spectral-domain optical coherence tomography.

atrophic tracts and streaks with decreased autofluorescence that correlate with the prior presence of subretinal fluid [82]. Interestingly, these tracts appear to follow gravity and typically show an outer border with increased autofluorescence [82]. NIR-AF tends to show more widespread abnormalities as compared to short-wavelength FAF [83]. Ultra-widefield FAF and indocyanine green angiography may reveal peripheral areas of previous or ongoing choroidal hyperpermeability and thereby assist in the diagnosis of central serous chorioretinopathy [84].

Inherited Retinal Diseases

Stargardt Disease

Stargardt disease (STGD1) represents the most common hereditary juvenile macular dystrophy and is caused by homozygous or compound heterozygous mutations in the *ABCA4* gene on chromosome 1p22. On FAF imaging, STGD1 is hallmarked by LF accumulation at the level of the RPE, which may be quantitatively measured using qAF or qualitatively recognized by the low detector sensitivity setting required for imaging [85]. Foveal or parafoveal atrophy typically results in lesions with decreased autofluorescence, while pisciform flecks exhibit typically increased

autofluorescence. The peripapillary region is usually spared from pathological abnormalities (peripapillary sparing).

Cideciyan et al. [85] proposed a model of disease sequence in STGD1 with 6 stages. Hereby, stage 1 represents normal structure and function of photoreceptors and RPE, as shown by normal parameters for rod and cone sensitivities, dark adaptation kinetics, and FAF intensity and texture. In stage 2, increased FAF intensity representing LF accumulation may be detected using FAF imaging. Stage 3 is characterized by an increase in FAF texture that could represent microscopic variations in the rates of LF accumulation or apical condensation of melanin granules observed in RPE cells laden with LF. Stage 4 is characterized by slowing of the rod and cone retinoid cycles and stage 5 by return of the FAF intensity to normal levels that may be secondary to the reduction in the number of viable RPE cells or reduced shedding of outer segment membrane as the photoreceptors degenerate. Stage 6 would indicate complete degeneration of photoreceptors and RPE [85].

Longitudinal short-wavelength FAF imaging revealed that the pisciform flecks with increased autofluorescence extend in a centrifugal direction from the fovea over time [86]. Hereby, longitudinal NIR-AF imaging also demonstrated centrifu-

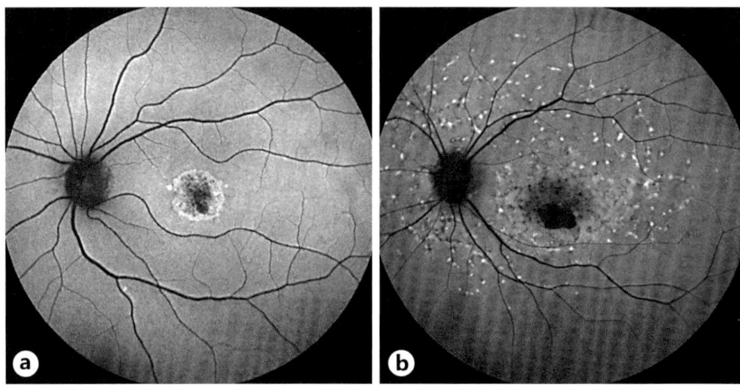

Fig. 10. Stargardt disease, the most common hereditary juvenile macular dystrophy caused by *ABCA4* mutations, may exhibit various phenotypic patterns. Patients hemizygous for p.G1961E (in *trans* with null) exhibit typically foveal atrophy with sparing of the peripheral retina (as shown in **a**). Other mutations result in a more widespread Stargardt phenotype characterized by foveal or parafoveal atrophy with pisciform flecks with increased autofluorescence. The peripapillary region is usually spared from pathological abnormalities (as shown in **b**).

gal lesion spread, but with fewer lesions with increased autofluorescence indicating a more transient increase in autofluorescence and more rapid decay [86]. Using NIR-AF imaging, it was also shown that the leading disease front shows an average centrifugal expansion rate of 2° per year [87]. This expansion rate of the disease front may hereby be accurately predicted based on the age and the former eccentricity of the leading disease front [87].

The FAF phenotype in STGD1 was also shown to correlate with the genotype (Fig. 10) [88]. Patients hemizygous for p.G1961E (in *trans* with null) typically exhibit foveal atrophy with sparing of the peripheral retina with an early or intermediate age at onset [88]. In contrast, patients hemizygous for p.R2030Q (in *trans* with null) were reported to commonly exhibit foveal sparing and well-defined RPE atrophy [88]. The latter phenotype ("fine granular with peripheral punctate spots") is also characteristic of so-called late-onset Stargardt disease that must be differentiated form GA secondary to AMD [69]. In comparison to GA secondary to AMD, late-onset Stargardt disease exhibits slower progression rates and significantly longer survival of the spared fovea [89]. Further, patients with STGD1 may not only exhibit areas of well-demarcated definitely decreased autofluorescence, but also well- and poorly demarcated questionably decreased autofluorescence that may be of prognostic relevance (Fig. 11) [90, 91].

Using qAF, it was not only possible to measure in vivo the increase in LF for different mutations, but also to measure LF levels in monoallelic carriers of *ABCA4* mutations (i.e., parents of patients) [92]. The results of two independent studies indicated that carriers of monoallelic *ABCA4* mutations show no abnormal LF accumulation [92–94]. However, in a small number of carriers, perifoveal fleck-like changes were visible [93]. The significance of this finding remains to be elucidated [93].

Analysis of fluorescence lifetimes in STGD1 patients revealed that the flecks with increased FAF signal are correlated with increased fluorescence lifetimes [95]. However, a subgroup of flecks with short lifetimes and no obvious changes in FAF intensity was also observed that appeared to precede flecks with increased FAF signal [95]. FLIO imaging may therefore provide additional prognostic information [95].

Retinitis Pigmentosa
Retinitis pigmentosa (RP) comprises a heterogeneous group of chronic genetic degenerative diseases of the retina that may be caused by a variety of genes. Loss of peripheral and night vision,

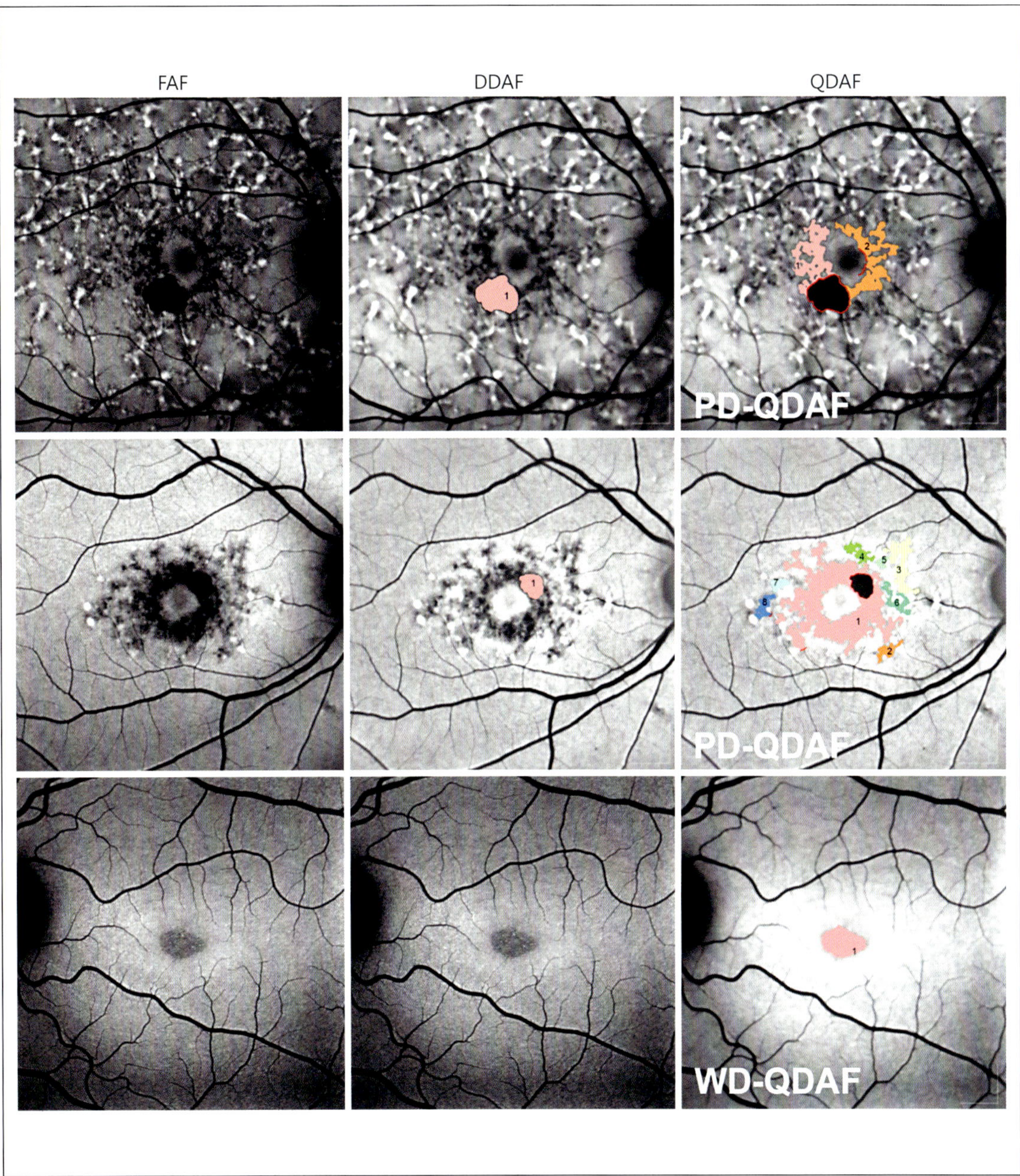

Fig. 11. In comparison with geographic atrophy secondary to age-related macular degeneration, Stargardt disease may not only exhibit areas of well-demarcated definitely decreased autofluorescence (WD-DDAF), but also areas of well- and poorly demarcated questionably decreased autofluorescence (WD-QDAF, PD-QDAF). These different types of atrophy may also be semiautomatically quantified using the RegionFinder™ as introduced by Schmitz-Valckenberg et al. [59] for geographic atrophy.

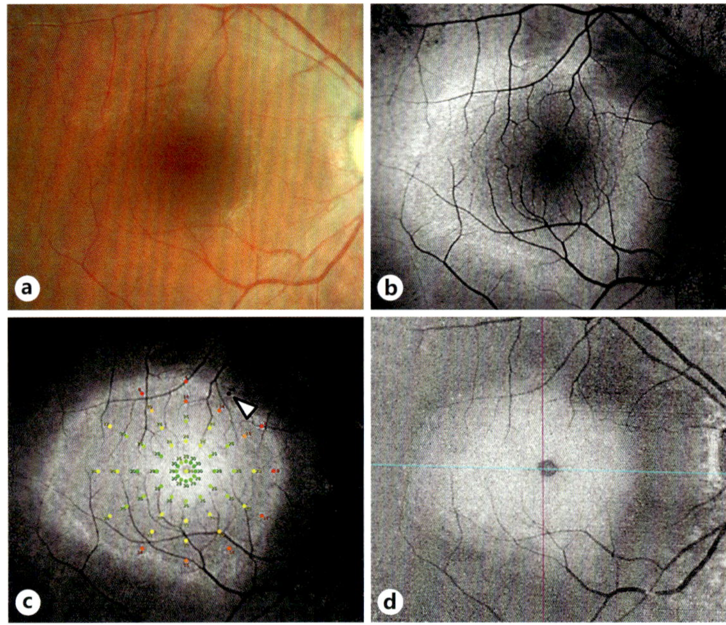

Fig. 12. On fundus autofluorescence imaging, a parafoveal ring with increased autofluorescence may be observable (Robson-Holder ring) in patients with retinitis pigmentosa. **a** Hereby, the ring of increased autofluorescence has typically no clear-cut correlate on color fundus photography. Commonly, the Robson-Holder ring is better visualized on near-infrared autofluorescence (**c**) images as compared to blue-light autofluorescence (**b**) images. The arrowhead shows a fundus perimetry test point with no measurable sensitivity indicating that the Robson-Holder ring precisely delineates the residual island of photoreceptors. Further, en face swept-source optical coherence tomography imaging (**d**) of the ellipsoid zone (band 2) confirms that the Robson-Holder ring correlates with intact photoreceptor outer segments.

which is rod-dependent, is usually among the first symptoms. Rhodopsin gene (*RHO*) mutations most commonly underlie autosomal-dominant RP, while mutations in the Usher's type 2 gene (*USH2A*) are most common in autosomal recessive RP. *RPGR* and *RP2* gene mutations underlie most commonly X-linked RP. On FAF imaging, a parafoveal ring with increased autofluorescence (Robson-Holder ring) may be observable (Fig. 12). Hereby, the pattern of electroretinography P50 amplitude correlates highly with the radius of the ring of increased autofluorescence [96]. Further, psychophysically it was observed that there is a gradient of sensitivity loss over the ring with severe threshold elevation outside the arc of the ring, indicating that the ring delineates the region of functionally preserved photoreceptors [97]. These discrete lines or rings of increased autofluorescence may also be observed in other retinal diseases – also with variable orientation, e.g. orientation along the retinal veins in pigmented paravenous chorioretinal atrophy [98].

The similar appearance suggests that these lines (or rings) in heterogeneous diseases including Leber congenital amaurosis, bull's eye maculopathy, X-linked retinoschisis, Best macular dystrophy, cone dystrophy, and cone-rod dystrophy may share common pathophysiological downstream pathways [98]. Using SD-OCT, Fleckenstein et al. [98] demonstrated that these discrete lines of increased autofluorescence correspond to the junctional zone between preserved outer retina and degenerated retina with the external limiting membrane in direct apposition to the RPE [99]. Further, it was confirmed that these rings represent not a relative but an absolute increase in the qAF signal of 15% as compared to eyes of similar age [100].

Best Vitelliform Dystrophy
Best vitelliform dystrophy is an inherited autosomal dominant early-onset dystrophy caused by mutations in the *BEST1* gene. All of the five disease stages of Best disease may be visualized using

FAF imaging: previtelliform stage (no or minimally increased autofluorescence), vitelliform lesion (well-circumscribed, homogenous increased autofluorescence), pseudohypopyon stage (gravitational layer of increased autofluorescence settling under iso-autofluorescent fluid), vitelliruptive stage (lesion with decreased autofluorescence bordered by condensations of increased autofluorescence) and the atrophic stage (well-defined area of decreased autofluorescence) [101]. The maximum qAF within the vitelliform lesion is elevated, and spectrofluorometric measurements are consistent with RPE LF [102]. In contrast, the nonlesional qAF is within normal limits, suggesting that no LF accumulation occurs in nonlesional fundus regions [102].

Pattern Dystrophies
Pattern dystrophies represent a heterogeneous group of late-onset, autosomal-dominant, symmetric macular dystrophies with a relatively good visual prognosis. However, over time, slow progressive central vision loss may occur.

Adult-onset foveomacular vitelliform dystrophy, the most common pattern dystrophy, has been associated with mutations in the *PRPH2*, *BEST1*, *IMPG1*, and *IMPG2* genes [103]. On FAF imaging, the central vitelliform lesion exhibits increased autofluorescence similar to Best vitelliform dystrophy [103–105].

Multifocal pattern dystrophy simulating Stargardt disease may also be caused by autosomal-dominant *PRPH2* mutations and shares significant phenotypic overlap with STGD1 [106, 107]. While both entities exhibit LF accumulation, *ABCA4* patients appear to have slightly higher qAF values than *PRPH2* patients [107]. Peripapillary sparing tends to be more common in *ABCA4* patients [106, 107]. Interestingly, other phenotypically mimicking pattern dystrophies without mutations in PRPH2/RDS or ABCA4 exhibit qAF levels within the normal range [107].

The other pattern dystrophies such as butterfly shaped pigment dystrophy, reticular dystrophy, and fundus pulverulentus show distinct abnormalities that tend to be more apparent on FAF imaging than on color fundus photography. However, studies substantiating the diagnostic benefit of FAF imaging for these diseases are missing.

Macular Telangiectasia Type 2
Macular telangiectasia type 2 (Mac Tel type 2) was first described by Gass in 1968 and refers to a bilateral disease characterized by abnormalities of capillaries of the fovea and perifoveal region ("Mac Tel area") associated with loss outer nuclear layers and ellipsoid zone [108–110]. Cystic cavitations and retinal thinning may become apparent, especially in the temporal parafovea. Interestingly, a progressive loss of luteal pigment is characteristic for Mac Tel type 2 [111, 112]. This may be evidenced by BAF images showing increased foveal FAF or by MPOD quantification using BAF and GAF imaging (Fig. 13). The loss of luteal pigment initially appears to be hereby more pronounced in the temporal parafovea compared to the nasal parafovea and more pronounced for zeaxanthin as compared to lutein [112]. A histological postmortem examination of an eye with Mac Tel type 2 confirmed the depletion of luteal pigment [113]. The topographically mapped MPOD allows for classification of Mac Tel type 2 into three classes: class 1 with a wedge-shaped loss of luteal pigment restricted to the temporal parafovea, class 2 with involvement of the fovea, and class 3 characterized by a pronounced loss within the oval "Mac Tel area" [114]. These classes correlate with the diseases stages as defined by Gass and Blodi [108]. Examination of very early disease manifestation in patients with asymmetric disease showed a severely reduced directional cone reflectance (Stiles-Crawford effect), asymmetric configuration of the foveal pit with focal temporal thinning most pronounced at 1° eccentricity, and topographically related, wedge-shaped MPOD reduction [115]. FAF and

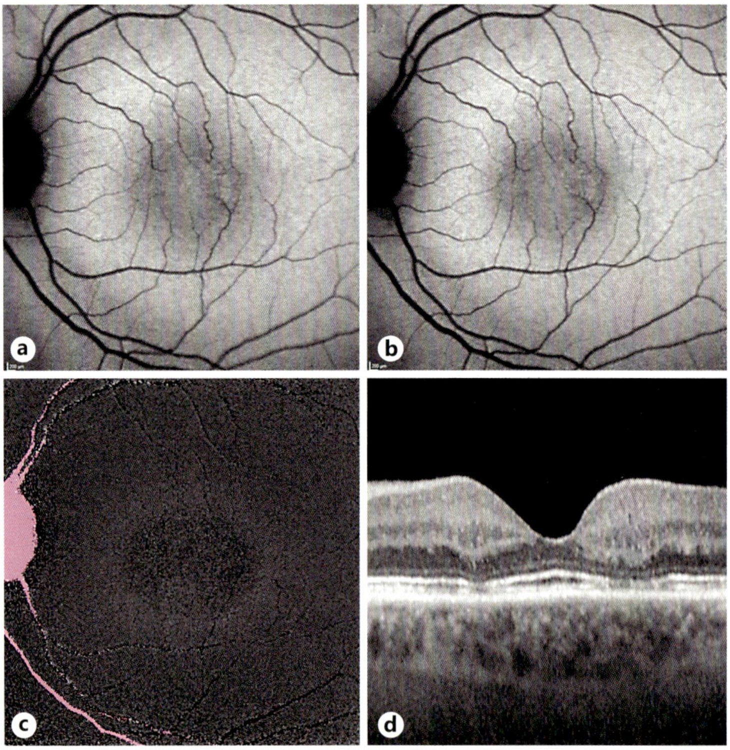

Fig. 13. Blue-light autofluorescence (BAF; **a**), green-light autofluorescence (GAF; **b**), macular pigment optical density (MPOD; **c**), and foveal horizontal spectral-domain optical coherence tomography (SD-OCT; **d**) of a patient with very early macular telangiectasia type 2 (Mac Tel type 2). The differences between the BAF and GAF images are minimal as indicated by the MPOD indicating the absence of luteal pigment – a characteristic finding for Mac Tel type 2. The SD-OCT reveals additional changes including irregularities of the ellipsoid zone (band 2) and thinning of the outer nuclear layer.

multimodal imaging appears to be promising for early identification of patients and affected family members [115].

Pseudoxanthoma Elasticum

Pseudoxanthoma elasticum (PXE) is an inherited systemic disease characterized by changes in the elastic tissue of the skin, eyes (Bruch's membrane), heart, and gastrointestinal system. It is caused by autosomal recessive mutations in the *ABCC6* gene [116]. The mineralization of Bruch's membrane may lead to various phenotypic alterations including angioid streaks, drusen of the optic nerve, peau d'orange, and comet-tail lesions (Fig. 14). In later stages, CNV and RPE atrophy may develop resulting in severe vision loss [116]. Interestingly, heterozygotes can show manifestations of the disease such as comet lesion and comet tail lesions (Fig. 14) [117]. Angioid streaks are typically visible as streaks of decreased autofluo-

rescence signal radiating from the optic disc. Comet-tail lesions may be seen in the midperiphery as spots with increased FAF signal [116]. CNV and RPE atrophy in PXE have an appearance similar to AMD [118, 119]. Reticular drusen were also shown to have a high prevalence in eyes of patients with PXE [120]. Although reticular pseudodrusen in patients with PXE occur at a younger age, their topographic distribution and phenotype were similar to reticular pseudodrusen associated with AMD [120]. This might hint towards common pathogenic downstream pathways in both diseases [120].

Choroideremia

Choroideremia (CHM), a rare hereditary retinal disease due to a mutation of the *CHM* gene located on the X chromosome, is characterized by an onset of night blindness during the first decade followed by progressive loss of peripheral vision

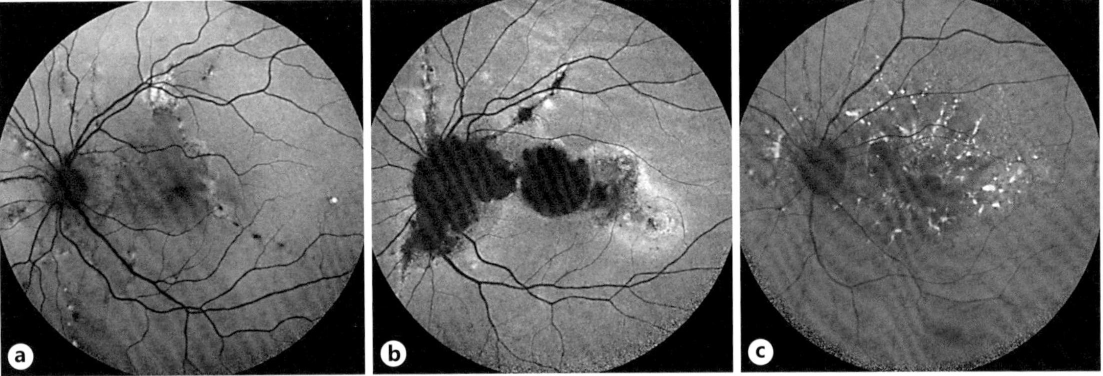

Fig. 14. a–c Wide-field 55° fundus autofluorescence (FAF) images of 3 patients with pseudoxanthoma elasticum. **a, b** Angioid streaks are clearly visible as streaks of decreased FAF signal radiating from the optic disc. **a** An exemplary comet-tail lesion is seen as a spot with increased FAF signal towards the temporal margin of the image. **b** A choroidal neovascularization can be diagnosed by blockage due to fibrosis and hemorrhages as well as increased FAF signal in areas with altered photoreceptor outer segments (c.f. "bleaching") that may indicate former presence of subretinal fluid. **c** This patient exhibits retinal pigment epithelium atrophy with phenotypic features similar to age-related macular degeneration.

[121]. CHM may result in total blindness when all remaining photoreceptors-islands have degenerated [121]. On FAF imaging, the remaining islands with preserved RPE appear as regions of normal or increased autofluorescence intensity due to LF accumulation, whereas areas with RPE atrophy are characterized by decreased autofluorescence [121, 122]. FAF imaging is especially of interest in CHM, since it allows for reproducible quantification of the residual autofluorescence and represents therefore a useful outcome measure [123]. Dysli et al. [124] demonstrated that autofluorescence lifetimes may additionally identify areas of remaining photoreceptors even in the absence of the RPE. Thus, the state of photoreceptors in patients with CHM may be assessed using FLIO in addition to the state of the residual RPE [124].

Fundus albipunctatus
Fundus albipunctatus is an autosomal recessive disorder of the *RDH5* gene, which encodes the 11-*cis* retinol dehydrogenase, an enzyme involved in the conversion of 11-*cis*-retinol to 11-*cis*-reti-

nal [125]. Most patients exhibit white dots extending into the midperiphery on fundus examination [125]. The defect in the visual cycle leads to night blindness and is characterized in FAF imaging by an extremely low signal indicating low concentrations of fluorophores such as LF [125].

Toxic Retinopathies

Chloroquine and Hydroxychloroquine Retinopathy
The use of the anti-inflammatory agent hydroxychloroquine (HCQ) will increase most likely following publication of the LUMINA study, which demonstrated a clear survival benefit of treated patients with systemic lupus erythematosus [126]. However, chloroquine (CQ) and HCQ may lead to retinopathy, especially in patients taking a daily HCQ dose greater than 5.0 mg/kg real weight [127]. Apart from a high daily and cumulative dose, concomitant renal disease and/or the use of tamoxifen represent major risk factors [127]. FAF imaging may allow for early detection of CQ/

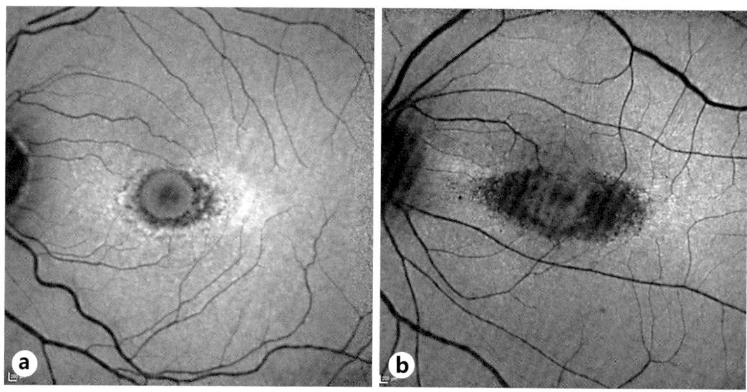

Fig. 15. Fundus autofluorescence imaging can be used for monitoring the status of the macula in patients at risk of various toxic retinopathies. **a, b** Two patients with chloroquine/hydroxychloroquine (CQ/HCQ) retinopathy. The disease typically manifests as a horseshoe-shaped atrophy of the outer retina and retinal pigment epithelium. If signs of CQ/HCQ are observed, the therapy with CQ/HCQ should be discontinued.

HCQ retinopathy showing a parafoveal ring of increased autofluorescence corresponding to photoreceptor damage (Fig. 15) [128]. In the later disease stage, parafoveally decreased autofluorescence due to RPE atrophy (bull's eye maculopathy) becomes apparent (Fig. 15) [128]. Besides SD-OCT and automated perimetry (10-2), FAF imaging and multifocal electroretinography were recommended as "additional useful screening tests" in the current American Academy of Ophthalmology recommendations on screening of CQ/HCQ retinopathy [127]. Noteworthy, patients of Asian origin may show early damage in a more peripheral pattern [127].

Other Toxic Retinopathies
FAF imaging is a helpful, fast, and noninvasive tool for monitoring the status of the macula in patients at risk of various toxic retinopathies.

Didanosine, a nucleoside reverse transcriptase inhibitor for HIV treatment, inhibits the synthesis of mitochondrial DNA [129]. Didanosine-induced retinal toxicity mirrors features of mitochondrial disorders with foveal sparing and patches of decreased autofluorescence corresponding to atrophy in the midperiphery [130–133]. These are typically surrounded by a mottled autofluorescence signal [130–133].

Deferoxamine-induced retinal toxicity, which is caused by a chelator used to treat iron overload, may show a variety of funduscopic manifestations including pigmentary abnormalities, vitelliform lesions, and bull's eye maculopathy [134]. In a prospective study, it was demonstrated that changes on FAF imaging were more apparent than on fundus photography [134].

References

1 Delori FC, Dorey CK, Staurenghi G, Arend O, Goger DG, Weiter JJ: In vivo fluorescence of the ocular fundus exhibits retinal pigment epithelium lipofuscin characteristics. Invest Ophthalmol Vis Sci 1995;36:718–729.

2 Dysli C, Wolf S, Berezin MY, Sauer L, Hammer M, Zinkernagel MS: Fluorescence lifetime imaging ophthalmoscopy. Prog Retin Eye Res 2017;60:120–143.

3 Weiter JJ, Delori FC, Wing GL, Fitch KA: Retinal pigment epithelial lipofuscin and melanin and choroidal melanin in human eyes. Invest Ophthalmol Vis Sci 1986;27:145–152.

4 Feeney-Burns L, Berman ER, Rothman H: Lipofuscin of human retinal pigment epithelium. Am J Ophthalmol 1980;90:783–791.

5 Wing GL, Blanchard GC, Weiter JJ: The topography and age relationship of lipofuscin concentration in the retinal pigment epithelium. Invest Ophthalmol Vis Sci 1978;17:601–607.

6 Sparrow JR, Boulton M: RPE lipofuscin and its role in retinal pathobiology. Exp Eye Res 2005;80:595–606.

7 Schmitz-Valckenberg S, Fleckenstein M, Scholl HPN, Holz FG: Fundus autofluorescence and progression of age-related macular degeneration. Surv Ophthalmol 2009;54:96–117.

8 Dorey CK, Wu G, Ebenstein D, Garsd A, Weiter JJ: Cell loss in the aging retina. Relationship to lipofuscin accumulation and macular degeneration. Invest Ophthalmol Vis Sci 1989;30:1691–1699.

9 Schutt F, Davies S, Kopitz J, Holz FG, Boulton ME: Photodamage to human RPE cells by A2-E, a retinoid component of lipofuscin. Invest Ophthalmol Vis Sci 2000;41:2303–2308.

10 Bergmann M, Schutt F, Holz FG, Kopitz J: Inhibition of the ATP-driven proton pump in RPE lysosomes by the major lipofuscin fluorophore A2-E may contribute to the pathogenesis of age-related macular degeneration. FASEB J 2004; 18:562–564.

11 Brunk UT, Wihlmark U, Wrigstad A, Roberg K, Nilsson SE: Accumulation of lipofuscin within retinal pigment epithelial cells results in enhanced sensitivity to photo-oxidation. Gerontology 1995; 41(suppl 2):201–212.

12 Hammer M, Richter S, Guehrs K-H, Schweitzer D: Retinal pigment epithelium cell damage by A2-E and its photo-derivatives. Mol Vis 2006;12:1348–1354.

13 Warrant EJ, Nilsson DE: Absorption of white light in photoreceptors. Vision Res 1998;38:195–207.

14 Theelen T, Berendschot TTJM, Boon CJF, Hoyng CB, Klevering BJ: Analysis of visual pigment by fundus autofluorescence. Exp Eye Res 2008;86:296–2304.

15 Snodderly DM, Brown PK, Delori FC, Auran JD: The macular pigment. I. Absorbance spectra, localization, and discrimination from other yellow pigments in primate retinas. Invest Ophthalmol Vis Sci 1984;25:660–673.

16 Whitehead AJ, Mares JA, Danis RP: Macular pigment: a review of current knowledge. Arch Ophthalmol 2006;124: 1038–1045.

17 Davies NP, Morland AB: Macular pigments: their characteristics and putative role. Prog Retin Eye Res 2004;23:533–559.

18 Delori FC, Goger DG, Hammond BR, Snodderly DM, Burns SA: Macular pigment density measured by autofluorescence spectrometry: comparison with reflectometry and heterochromatic flicker photometry. J Opt Soc Am A Opt Image Sci Vis 2001;18:1212–1230.

19 Wolf-Schnurrbusch UE, Wittwer VV, Ghanem R, et al: Blue light versus green light autofluorescence: lesion size of areas with geographic atrophy. Invest Ophthalmol Vis Sci 2011;52:9497–9502.

20 Pfau M, Goerdt L, Schmitz-Valckenberg S, et al: Green-light autofluorescence versus combined blue-light autofluorescence and near-infrared reflectance imaging in geographic atrophy secondary to age-related macular degeneration. Invest Ophthalmol Vis Sci 2017; 58:BIO121–BIO130.

21 Keilhauer CN, Delori FC: Near-infrared autofluorescence imaging of the fundus: visualization of ocular melanin. Invest Ophthalmol Vis Sci 2006;47:3556–3564.

22 Weinberger AWA, Lappas A, Kirschkamp T, et al: Fundus near infrared fluorescence correlates with fundus near infrared reflectance. Invest Ophthalmol Vis Sci 2006;47:3098–3108.

23 Kellner U, Kellner S, Weinitz S: Fundus autofluorescence (488 NM) and near-infrared autofluorescence (787 NM) visualize different retinal pigment epithelium alterations in patients with age-related macular degeneration. Retina 2010;30:6–15.

24 Gibbs D, Cideciyan AV, Jacobson SG, Williams DS: Retinal pigment epithelium defects in humans and mice with mutations in MYO7A: imaging melanosome-specific autofluorescence. Invest Ophthalmol Vis Sci 2009;50:4386–4393.

25 Schmitz-Valckenberg S, Lara D, Nizari S, et al: Localisation and significance of in vivo near-infrared autofluorescent signal in retinal imaging. Br J Ophthalmol 2011;95:1134–1139.

26 Delori FC, Fleckner MR, Goger DG, Weiter JJ, Dorey CK: Autofluorescence distribution associated with drusen in age-related macular degeneration. Invest Ophthalmol Vis Sci 2000;41:496–504.

27 Spaide RF: Fundus autofluorescence and age-related macular degeneration. Ophthalmology 2003;110:392–399.

28 Webb RH, Hughes GW, Delori FC: Confocal scanning laser ophthalmoscope. Appl Opt 1987;26:1492–1499.

29 von Rückmann, Fitzke FW, Bird C, von Ruckmann A, Fitzke FW, Bird C: Distribution of fundus autofluorescence with a scanning laser ophthalmoscope. Br J Ophthalmol 1995;79:407–412.

30 Oishi M, Oishi A, Ogino K, et al: Wide-field fundus autofluorescence abnormalities and visual function in patients with cone and cone-rod dystrophies. Invest Ophthalmol Vis Sci 2014;55:3572–3577.

31 Witmer MT, Kozbial A, Daniel S, Kiss S: Peripheral autofluorescence findings in age-related macular degeneration. Acta Ophthalmol 2012;90:e428–e433.

32 Tan CS, Heussen F, Sadda SR: Peripheral autofluorescence and clinical findings in neovascular and non-neovascular age-related macular degeneration. Ophthalmology 2013;120:1271–1277.

33 Duisdieker V, Fleckenstein M, Zilkens KM, Steinberg JS, Holz FG, Schmitz-Valckenberg S: Long-term follow-up of fundus autofluorescence imaging using wide-field scanning laser ophthalmoscopy. Ophthalmologica 2015;234:218–226.

34 Delori F, Greenberg JP, Woods RL, et al: Quantitative measurements of autofluorescence with the scanning laser ophthalmoscope. Invest Ophthalmol Vis Sci 2011;52:9379–9390.

35 Greenberg JP, Duncker T, Woods RL, Smith RT, Sparrow JR, Delori FC: Quantitative fundus autofluorescence in healthy eyes. Invest Ophthalmol Vis Sci 2013;54:5684–5693.

36 Schweitzer D, Kolb A, Hammer M: Autofluorescence lifetime measurements in images of the human ocular fundus. Diagn Opt Spectrosc Biomed Proc SPIE 2001;4432:29–39.

37 Schweitzer D, Kolb A, Hammer M, Thamm E: Basic investigations for 2-dimensional time-resolved fluorescence measurements at the fundus. Int Ophthalmol 2001;23:399–404.

38 Schweitzer D, Kolb A, Hammer M, Anders R: Zeitaufgelöste Messung der Autofluoreszenz. Ophthalmologe 2002;99:774–779.

39 Lim LS, Mitchell P, Seddon JM, Holz FG, Wong TY: Age-related macular degeneration. Lancet 2012;379:1728–1738.

40 Bindewald A, Bird AC, Dandekar SSS, et al: Classification of fundus autofluorescence patterns in early age-related macular disease. Invest Ophthalmol Vis Sci 2005;46:3309–3314.

41 Boon CJF, van de Ven JPH, Hoyng CB, den Hollander AI, Klevering BJ: Cuticular drusen: stars in the sky. Prog Retin Eye Res 2013;37:90–113.

42 Mimoun G, Soubrane G, Coscas G: Macular drusen (in French). J Fr Ophtalmol 1990;13:511–530.

43 Schmitz-Valckenberg S, Steinberg JS, Fleckenstein M, Visvalingam S, Brinkmann CK, Holz FG: Combined confocal scanning laser ophthalmoscopy and spectral-domain optical coherence tomography imaging of reticular drusen associated with age-related macular degeneration. Ophthalmology 2010;117: 1169–1176.

44 Zweifel SA, Spaide RF, Curcio CA, Malek G, Imamura Y: Reticular pseudodrusen are subretinal drusenoid deposits. Ophthalmology 2010;117:303–12.e1.

45 Cohen SY, Dubois L, Tadayoni R, Delahaye-Mazza C, Debibie C, Quentel G: Prevalence of reticular pseudodrusen in age-related macular degeneration with newly diagnosed choroidal neovascularisation. Br J Ophthalmol 2007;91: 354–359.

46 Smith RT, Chan JK, Busuoic M, Sivagnanavel V, Bird AC, Chong NV: Autofluorescence characteristics of early, atrophic, and high-risk fellow eyes in age-related macular degeneration. Invest Ophthalmol Vis Sci 2006;47:5495–5504.

47 Pumariega NM, Smith RT, Sohrab MA, Letien V, Souied EH: A prospective study of reticular macular disease. Ophthalmology 2011;118:1619–1625.

48 Finger RP, Wu Z, Luu CD, et al: Reticular pseudodrusen: a risk factor for geographic atrophy in fellow eyes of individuals with unilateral choroidal neovascularization. Ophthalmology 2014;121:1252–1256.

49 Suzuki M, Sato T, Spaide RF: Pseudodrusen subtypes as delineated by multimodal imaging of the fundus. Am J Ophthalmol 2014;157:1005–1012.

50 Batioglu F, Demirel S, Ozmert E, Oguz YG, Ozyol P: Autofluorescence patterns as a predictive factor for neovascularization. Optom Vis Sci 2014;91:950–955.

51 Einbock W, Moessner A, Schnurrbusch UEK, Holz FG, Wolf S: Changes in fundus autofluorescence in patients with age-related maculopathy. Correlation to visual function: a prospective study. Graefes Arch Clin Exp Ophthalmol 2005;243:300–305.

52 Gliem M, Müller PL, Finger RP, McGuinness MB, Holz FG, Charbel Issa P: Quantitative fundus autofluorescence in early and intermediate age-related macular degeneration. JAMA Ophthalmol 2016;134:817–824.

53 Dysli C, Fink R, Wolf S, Zinkernagel MS: Fluorescence lifetimes of drusen in age-related macular degeneration. Invest Ophthalmol Vis Sci 2017;58:4856–4862.

54 von Ruckmann A, Fitzke FW, Bird AC: In vivo fundus autofluorescence in macular dystrophies. Arch Ophthalmol 1997;115:609–615.

55 Holz FG, Bellmann C, Margaritidis M, Schütt F, Otto TP, Völcker HE: Patterns of increased in vivo fundus autofluorescence in the junctional zone of geographic atrophy of the retinal pigment epithelium associated with age-related macular degeneration. Graefes Arch Clin Exp Ophthalmol 1999;237:145–152.

56 Dreyhaupt J, Mansmann U, Pritsch M, Dolar-Szczasny J, Bindewald A, Holz FG: Modelling the natural history of geographic atrophy in patients with age-related macular degeneration. Ophthalmic Epidemiol 2005;12:353–362.

57 Holz FG, Bindewald-Wittich A, Fleckenstein M, Dreyhaupt J, Scholl HPN, Schmitz-Valckenberg S: Progression of geographic atrophy and impact of fundus autofluorescence patterns in age-related macular degeneration. Am J Ophthalmol 2007;143:463–472.

58 Deckert A, Schmitz-Valckenberg S, Jorzik J, Bindewald A, Holz FG, Mansmann U: Automated analysis of digital fundus autofluorescence images of geographic atrophy in advanced age-related macular degeneration using confocal scanning laser ophthalmoscopy (cSLO). BMC Ophthalmol 2005;5:8.

59 Schmitz-Valckenberg S, Brinkmann CK, Alten F, et al: Semiautomated image processing method for identification and quantification of geographic atrophy in age-related macular degeneration. Invest Ophthalmol Vis Sci 2011;52: 7640–7646.

60 Lindner M, Böker A, Mauschitz MM, et al: Directional kinetics of geographic atrophy progression in age-related macular degeneration with foveal sparing. Ophthalmology 2015;122:1356–1365.

61 Lee N, Laine A, Smith R: A hybrid segmentation approach for geographic atrophy in fundus auto-fluorescence images for diagnosis of age-related macular degeneration. Conf Proc IEEE Eng Med Biol Soc 2007;2007:4965–4968.

62 Hu Z, Medioni GG, Hernandez M, Hariri A, Wu X, Sadda SR: Segmentation of the geographic atrophy in spectral-domain optical coherence tomography and fundus autofluorescence images. Invest Ophthalmol Vis Sci 2013;54:8375–8383.

63 Holz FG, Sadda SR, Staurenghi G, et al: Imaging protocols in clinical studies in advanced age-related macular degeneration: recommendations from Classification of Atrophy Consensus Meetings. Ophthalmology 2017;124:464–478.

64 Wu Z, Luu CD, Ayton LN, et al: Fundus autofluorescence characteristics of nascent geographic atrophy in age-related macular degeneration. Invest Ophthalmol Vis Sci 2015;56:1546–1552.

65 Schmitz-Valckenberg S, Bindewald-Wittich A, Dolar-Szczasny J, et al: Correlation between the area of increased autofluorescence surrounding geographic atrophy and disease progression in patients with AMD. Invest Ophthalmol Vis Sci 2006;47:2648–2654.

66 Batioglu F, Oguz YG, Demirel S, Özmert E: Geographic atrophy progression in eyes with age-related macular degeneration: role of fundus autofluorescence patterns, fellow eye and baseline atrophy area. Ophthalmic Res 2014;52:53–59.

67 Jeong YJ, Hong IH, Chung JK, Kim KL, Kim HK, Park SP: Predictors for the progression of geographic atrophy in patients with age-related macular degeneration: fundus autofluorescence study with modified fundus camera. Eye 2014;28:209–218.

68 Schmitz-Valckenberg S, Sahel JA, Danis R, et al: Natural history of geographic atrophy progression secondary to age-related macular degeneration (Geographic Atrophy Progression Study). Ophthalmology 2016;123:361–368.

69 Fritsche LG, Fleckenstein M, Fiebig BS, et al: A subgroup of age-related macular degeneration is associated with mono-allelic sequence variants in the *ABCA4* gene. Invest Opthalmol Vis Sci 2012;53:2112.

70 Fleckenstein M, Grassmann F, Lindner M, et al: Distinct genetic risk profile of the rapidly progressing diffuse-trickling subtype of geographic atrophy in age-related macular degeneration (AMD). Invest Ophthalmol Vis Sci 2016;57:2463–2471.

71 Fleckenstein M, Schmitz-Valckenberg S, Martens C, et al: Fundus autofluorescence and spectral-domain optical coherence tomography characteristics in a rapidly progressing form of geographic atrophy. Invest Ophthalmol Vis Sci 2011;52:3761–3766.

72 Vaclavik V, Vujosevic S, Dandekar SS, Bunce C, Peto T, Bird AC: Autofluorescence imaging in age-related macular degeneration complicated by choroidal neovascularization: a prospective study. Ophthalmology 2008;115:342–346.

73 McBain VA, Townend J, Lois N: Fundus autofluorescence in exudative age-related macular degeneration. Br J Ophthalmol 2007;91:491–496.

74 Camacho N, Barteselli G, Nezgoda JT, et al: Significance of the hyperautofluorescent ring associated with choroidal neovascularisation in eyes undergoing anti-VEGF therapy for wet age-related macular degeneration. Br J Ophthalmol 2015;99:1277–1283.

75 Heimes B, Lommatzsch A, Zeimer M, et al: Foveal RPE autofluorescence as a prognostic factor for anti-VEGF therapy in exudative AMD. Graefes Arch Clin Exp Ophthalmol 2008;246:1229–1234.

76 Sarraf D, Joseph A, Rahimy E: Retinal pigment epithelial tears in the era of intravitreal pharmacotherapy: risk factors, pathogenesis, prognosis and treatment (an American Ophthalmological Society thesis). Trans Am Ophthalmol Soc 2014;112:142–159.

77 Karadimas P, Paleokastritis GP, Bouzas EA: Fundus autofluorescence imaging findings in retinal pigment epithelial tear. Eur J Ophthalmol 2006;16:767–769.

78 Mendis R, Lois N: Fundus autofluorescence in patients with retinal pigment epithelial (RPE) tears: an in vivo evaluation of RPE resurfacing. Graefes Arch Clin Exp Ophthalmol 2014;252:1059–1063.

79 Caramoy A, Fauser S, Kirchhof B: Fundus autofluorescence and spectral-domain optical coherence tomography findings suggesting tissue remodelling in retinal pigment epithelium tear. Br J Ophthalmol 2012;96:1211–1216.

80 Vujosevic S, Casciano M, Pilotto E, Boccassini B, Varano M, Midena E: Diabetic macular edema: fundus autofluorescence and functional correlations. Invest Ophthalmol Vis Sci 2011;52:442–448.

81 Bessho K, Gomi F, Harino S, et al: Macular autofluorescence in eyes with cystoid macula edema, detected with 488 nm-excitation but not with 580 nm-excitation. Graefes Arch Clin Exp Ophthalmol 2009;247:729–734.

82 Spaide RF, Klancnik JMJ: Fundus autofluorescence and central serous chorioretinopathy. Ophthalmology 2005;112:825–833.

83 Zhang P, Wang H-Y, Zhang Z-F, et al: Fundus autofluorescence in central serous chorioretinopathy: association with spectral-domain optical coherence tomography and fluorescein angiography. Int J Ophthalmol 2015;8:1003–1007.

84 Pang CE, Shah VP, Sarraf D, Freund KB: Ultra-widefield imaging with autofluorescence and indocyanine green angiography in central serous chorioretinopathy. Am J Ophthalmol 2014;158:362–371.e2.

85 Cideciyan A V, Aleman TS, Swider M, et al: Mutations in ABCA4 result in accumulation of lipofuscin before slowing of the retinoid cycle: a reappraisal of the human disease sequence. Hum Mol Genet 2004;13:525–534.

86 Cukras CA, Wong WT, Caruso R, Cunningham D, Zein W, Sieving PA: Centrifugal expansion of fundus autofluorescence patterns in Stargardt disease over time. Arch Ophthalmol 2012;130:171–179.

87 Cideciyan AV, Swider M, Schwartz SB, Stone EM, Jacobson SG: Predicting progression of ABCA4-associated retinal degenerations based on longitudinal measurements of the leading disease front. Invest Ophthalmol Vis Sci 2015;56:5946–5955.

88 Fakin A, Robson AG, Chiang JP-W, et al: The effect on retinal structure and function of 15 specific ABCA4 mutations: a detailed examination of 82 hemizygous patients. Invest Ophthalmol Vis Sci 2016;57:5963–5973.

89 Lindner M, Lambertus S, Mauschitz MM, et al: Differential disease progression in atrophic age-related macular degeneration and late-onset Stargardt disease. Invest Opthalmol Vis Sci 2017;58:1001.

90 Kuehlewein L, Hariri AH, Ho A, et al: Comparison of manual and semiautomated fundus autofluorescence analysis of macular atrophy in Stargardt disease phenotype. Retina 2016;36:1216–1221.

91 Strauss RW, Muñoz B, Ho A, et al: Incidence of atrophic lesions in Stargardt disease in the progression of atrophy secondary to Stargardt disease (ProgStar) Study. JAMA Ophthalmol 2017;53:841–852.

92 Burke TR, Duncker T, Woods RL, et al: Quantitative fundus autofluorescence in recessive Stargardt disease. Invest Ophthalmol Vis Sci 2014;55:2841–2852.

93 Duncker T, Stein GE, Lee W, et al: Quantitative fundus autofluorescence and optical coherence tomography in ABCA4 carriers. Invest Ophthalmol Vis Sci 2015;56:7274–7285.

94 Muller PL, Gliem M, Mangold E, et al: Monoallelic ABCA4 mutations appear insufficient to cause retinopathy: a quantitative autofluorescence study. Invest Ophthalmol Vis Sci 2015;56:8179–8186.

95 Dysli C, Wolf S, Hatz K, Zinkernagel MS: Fluorescence lifetime imaging in Stargardt Disease: potential marker for disease progression. Invest Ophthalmol Vis Sci 2016;57:832–841.

96 Robson AG, El-Amir A, Bailey C, et al: Pattern ERG correlates of abnormal fundus autofluorescence in patients with retinitis pigmentosa and normal visual acuity. Invest Ophthalmol Vis Sci 2003;44:3544–3550.

97 Robson AG, Egan CA, Luong VA, Bird AC, Holder GE, Fitzke FW: Comparison of fundus autofluorescence with photopic and scotopic fine-matrix mapping in patients with retinitis pigmentosa and normal visual acuity. Invest Ophthalmol Vis Sci 2004;45:4119–4125.

98 Fleckenstein M, Charbel Issa P, Fuchs HA, et al: Discrete arcs of increased fundus autofluorescence in retinal dystrophies and functional correlate on microperimetry. Eye 2009;23:567–775.

99 Robson AG, Tufail A, Fitzke F, et al: Serial imaging and structure-function correlates of high-density rings of fundus autofluorescence in retinitis pigmentosa. Retina 2011;31:1670–1679.

100 Schuerch K, Woods RL, Lee W, et al: Quantifying fundus autofluorescence in patients with retinitis pigmentosa. Invest Ophthalmol Vis Sci 2017;58:1843–1855.

101 Querques G, Zerbib J, Georges A, et al: Multimodal analysis of the progression of best vitelliform macular dystrophy. Mol Vis 2014;20:575–592.

102 Duncker T, Greenberg JP, Ramachandran R, et al: Quantitative fundus autofluorescence and optical coherence tomography in best vitelliform macular dystrophy. Invest Ophthalmol Vis Sci 2014;55:1471–1482.

103 Boon CJF, Klevering BJ, den Hollander AI, et al: Clinical and genetic heterogeneity in multifocal vitelliform dystrophy. Arch Ophthalmol 2007;125:1100–1106.

104 Renner AB, Tillack H, Kraus H, et al: Morphology and functional characteristics in adult vitelliform macular dystrophy. Retina 2004;24:929–939.

105 Querques G, Forte R, Querques L, Massamba N, Souied EH: Natural course of adult-onset foveomacular vitelliform dystrophy: a spectral-domain optical coherence tomography analysis. Am J Ophthalmol 2011;152:304–313.

106 Boon CJ, van Schooneveld MJ, den Hollander AI, et al: Mutations in the peripherin/RDS gene are an important cause of multifocal pattern dystrophy simulating STGD1/fundus flavimaculatus. Br J Ophthalmol 2007;91:1504–1511.

107 Duncker T, Tsang SH, Woods RL, et al: Quantitative fundus autofluorescence and optical coherence tomography in PRPH2/RDS- and ABCA4-associated disease exhibiting phenotypic overlap. Invest Ophthalmol Vis Sci 2015;56:3159–3170.

108 Gass JD, Blodi BA: Idiopathic juxtafoveolar retinal telangiectasis. Update of classification and follow-up study. Ophthalmology 1993;100:1536–1546.

109 Hutton WL, Snyder WB, Fuller D, Vaiser A: Focal parafoveal retinal telangiectasis. Arch Ophthalmol 1978;96:1362–1367.

110 Gass JDM: Stereoscopic Atlas of Macular Diseases: Diagnosis and Treatment, ed 4. St Louis, Mosby, 1997.

111 Helb H-M, Charbel Issa P, van der Veen RLP, Berendschot TTJM, Scholl HPN, Holz FG: Abnormal macular pigment distribution in type 2 idiopathic macular telangiectasia. Retina 2008;28:808–816.

112 Charbel Issa P, van der Veen RLP, Stijfs A, Holz FG, Scholl HPN, Berendschot TTJM: Quantification of reduced macular pigment optical density in the central retina in macular telangiectasia type 2. Exp Eye Res 2009;89:25–31.

113 Powner MB, Gillies MC, Tretiach M, et al: Perifoveal muller cell depletion in a case of macular telangiectasia type 2. Ophthalmology 2010;117:2407–2416.

114 Zeimer MB, Padge B, Heimes B, Pauleikhoff D: Idiopathic macular telangiectasia type 2: distribution of macular pigment and functional investigations. Retina 2010;30:586–595.

115 Charbel Issa P, Heeren TFC, Kupitz EH, Holz FG, Berendschot TTJM: Very early disease manifestations of macular telangiectasia type 2. Retina 2016;36:524–534.

116 Gliem M, Zaeytijd JD, Finger RP, Holz FG, Leroy BP, Charbel Issa P: An update on the ocular phenotype in patients with pseudoxanthoma elasticum. Front Genet 2013;4:14.

117 De Zaeytijd J, Vanakker OM, Coucke PJ, De Paepe A, De Laey J-J, Leroy BP: Added value of infrared, red-free and autofluorescence fundus imaging in pseudoxanthoma elasticum. Br J Ophthalmol 2010;94:479–486.

118 Gliem M, Muller PL, Birtel J, Hendig D, Holz FG, Charbel Issa P: Frequency, phenotypic characteristics and progression of atrophy associated with a diseased Bruch's membrane in pseudoxanthoma elasticum. Invest Ophthalmol Vis Sci 2016;57:3323–3330.

119 Charbel Issa P, Finger RP, Gotting C, Hendig D, Holz FG, Scholl HPN: Centrifugal fundus abnormalities in pseudoxanthoma elasticum. Ophthalmology 2010;117:1406–1414.

120 Gliem M, Hendig D, Finger RP, Holz FG, Charbel Issa P: Reticular pseudodrusen associated with a diseased Bruch membrane in pseudoxanthoma elasticum. JAMA Ophthalmol 2015;133:581–588.

121 Zinkernagel MS, MacLaren RE: Recent advances and future prospects in choroideremia. Clin Ophthalmol 2015;9:2195–2200.

122 Syed R, Sundquist SM, Ratnam K, et al: High-resolution images of retinal structure in patients with choroideremia. Invest Ophthalmol Vis Sci 2013;54:950–961.

123 Jolly JK, Edwards TL, Moules J, Groppe M, Downes SM, MacLaren RE: A qualitative and quantitative assessment of fundus autofluorescence patterns in patients with choroideremia. Invest Ophthalmol Vis Sci 2016;57:4498–4503.

124 Dysli C, Wolf S, Tran HV, Zinkernagel MS: Autofluorescence lifetimes in patients with choroideremia identify photoreceptors in areas with retinal pigment epithelium atrophy. Invest Ophthalmol Vis Sci 2016;57:6714–6721.

125 Sergouniotis PI, Sohn EH, Li Z, et al: Phenotypic variability in RDH5 retinopathy (fundus albipunctatus). Ophthalmology 2011;118:1661–1670.

126 Alarcon GS, McGwin G, Bertoli AM, et al: Effect of hydroxychloroquine on the survival of patients with systemic lupus erythematosus: data from LUMINA, a multiethnic US cohort (LUMINA L). Ann Rheum Dis 2007;66:1168–1172.

127 Marmor MF, Kellner U, Lai TYY, Melles RB, Mieler WF: Recommendations on screening for chloroquine and hydroxychloroquine retinopathy (2016 revision). Ophthalmology 2016;123:1386–1394.

128 Kellner U, Renner AB, Tillack H: Fundus autofluorescence and mfERG for early detection of retinal alterations in patients using chloroquine/hydroxychloroquine. Invest Ophthalmol Vis Sci 2006;47:3531–3538.

129 Wang H, Lemire BD, Cass CE, et al: Zidovudine and dideoxynucleosides deplete wild-type mitochondrial DNA levels and increase deleted mitochondrial DNA levels in cultured Kearns-Sayre syndrome fibroblasts. Biochim Biophys Acta 1996;1316:51–59.

130 Whitcup SM, Dastgheib K, Nussenblatt RB, Walton RC, Pizzo PA, Chan CC: A clinicopathologic report of the retinal lesions associated with didanosine. Arch Ophthalmol 1994;112:1594–1598.

131 Gabrielian A, MacCumber MM, Kukuyev A, Mitsuyasu R, Holland GN, Sarraf D: Didanosine-associated retinal toxicity in adults infected with human immunodeficiency virus. JAMA Ophthalmol 2013;131:255–259.

132 Pinto R, Lino S, Nogueira V, Fonseca A, Ornelas C: A woman with didanosine retinopathy and non-cirrhotic portal hypertension. Int J STD AIDS 2013;24:247–249.

133 Cobo J, Ruiz MF, Figueroa MS, et al: Retinal toxicity associated with didanosine in HIV-infected adults. AIDS 1996;10:1297–1300.

134 Viola F, Barteselli G, Dell'arti L, et al: Abnormal fundus autofluorescence results of patients in long-term treatment with deferoxamine. Ophthalmology 2012;119:1693–1700.

Prof. Dr. Frank G. Holz
Department of Ophthalmology, University of Bonn
Ernst-Abbe-Strasse 2
DE–53127 Bonn (Germany)
E-Mail Frank.Holz@ukbonn.de

Cunha-Vaz J, Koh A (eds): Imaging Techniques.
ESASO Course Series. Basel, Karger, 2018, vol 10, pp 88–101 (DOI: 10.1159/000487414)

Noninvasive Multimodal Imaging of Diabetic Retinopathy

Inês Marques · Luís Mendes · José Cunha-Vaz

AIBILI – Association for Innovation and Biomedical Research on Light and Image, Coimbra, Portugal

Abstract

The abnormalities seen in diabetic retinopathy (DR) can be split into three categories: findings resulting from structural retinal neurodegeneration, findings resulting from leaking microvasculature, and findings resulting from microvascular alterations with ischemia. Noninvasive multimodal imaging, making use of different imaging techniques such as fundus color photography (CFP) and optical coherence tomography (OCT), allows for better characterization of diabetic retinal disease. With the advent of spectral-domain OCT and OCT angiography we may, for the first time, look at the different components of diabetic retinal damage – retinal neurodegeneration, edema, and microvascular changes – in a multimodal approach. The variables that represent microvascular changes (vessel density of superficial retina plexus and deep retinal plexus, foveal avascular zone area and circu-larity, and microaneurysm turnover), retinal neurodegeneration (thinning of the retinal nerve fiber layer and ganglion cell layer + inner plexiform layers), and retinal edema (increased thickness of the inner nuclear and outer plexiform layers of the retina) show a wide range of values between different eyes in each nonproliferative DR ETDRS (Early Treatment Diabetic Retinopathy Study) level, demonstrating that there are very different degrees of microvascular damage, neurodegenerative changes, and edema in different eyes in the same retinopathy grade. This conclusion supports the concept of three major phenotypes of retinal disease in type 2 diabetes. This noninvasive approach allows for repeated examinations in longitudinal studies, helping in finding specific progression patterns to personalize treatment and follow-up.
© 2018 S. Karger AG, Basel

Diabetic retinopathy (DR) is one of the most challenging problems facing ophthalmological research. Its incidence continues to increase all over the world, so that it remains one of the most frequent causes of blindness [1, 2].

Ashton, who has contributed so extensively to our knowledge of DR, remarked in 1974 that "we must continue to look for more fundamental scientific investigations and at the same time develop new ways of examining the diabetic retina in an effort to unravel the still unsolved mysteries of diabetic retinopathy" [3]. The recent advent of different imaging modalities has opened new perspectives, and multimodal imaging of the diabetic retina in different stages of its progress is timely.

In 1978, Cunha-Vaz [4] reviewed the pathology of DR and other vascular retinopathies using post-mortem injection methods, a variety of stains, and the digestion technique using a truly multimodal approach. Light microscopic examination of retinal "digests" is particularly appropriate to study alterations in the retinal vascular bed. From this study, a well-defined pattern of disease was observed to occur in DR. The results suggested that changes are initially confined to the small vessels in the form of endothelial proliferation, pericyte loss, rare microaneurysms (MAs), and signs of impending cellular degeneration in a few vascular branches [4]. These initial lesions are focal and located preferentially at the posterior pole of the retina. The endothelial proliferation and MAs appeared to be confined to the venous side of the retinal circulation, whereas at this stage, endothelial degeneration appears better identified in capillaries on the arterial side of the circulation.

With the progression of the disease, the capillaries on the arterial side of the retinal circulation show increased cell loss and closure. Simultaneously, on the venous side of the circulation, there is an increase in the number of MAs. As the areas of capillary closure enlarge, they are seen to be traversed by a few enlarged capillaries, which appear to act as arteriovenous shunts, receiving the blood diverted from the surrounding closed capillary net. These observations are summarized in Table 1.

Are these lesions specific for diabetes? Examination of other vascular retinopathies emphasizes the probable importance of local factors and shows that the lesions described in DR are shared by a wide variety of apparently unrelated diseases.

An abnormality of the blood-retinal barrier, demonstrated both by vitreous fluorometry and fluorescein angiography, is also an early finding both in human and experimental diabetes [5, 6]. The alteration of the blood-retinal barrier is well demonstrated by fluorescein leakage and it is accepted that it leads to the development of retinal edema.

DR has been considered a microvascular complication of diabetes clinically identified by changes produced either due to progressive cell degeneration and vasoregression or due to abnormalities of the blood-retinal barrier, limiting the diagnostic and therapeutic focus to the vascular system. However, it is now accepted that diabetic retinal disease involves the neuronal as well as the vascular compartments [7]. Attempts have been made to identify functional changes of the retina that may precede MAs, such as blood flow changes, but the results have been contradictory mainly because of technical problems and lack of reliable methodology [8, 9]. Subtle changes in microvascular hemodynamics are expected to be one of the earliest changes to occur in DR.

Vision loss is associated with the two major complications of DR, clinically significant macular edema and proliferative DR, and does not occur before these complications develop [10]. Those complications are the clinically meaningful outcomes. This concept is crucial. There is, therefore, a clear need to identify biomarkers of diabetic retinal disease progression that predict the development of these late clinically significant outcomes directly associated with vision loss.

Table 1. Evolution of retinal vascular lesions in diabetes

Stage	Ophthalmoscopy	Pathology, small vessels	
		venous side	arterial side
0	–	?	
1 – initial	Rare aneurysm	Endothelial proliferation ++ Aneurysm ++	Endothelial degeneration +
2 – intermediate	Numerous aneurysms Hemorrhages Exudate	Endothelial proliferation ++ Aneurysm ++	Endothelial degeneration ++ Focal capillary closure
3 – advanced	Same lesions as in stage 2 Large hemorrhages Venous beading	Endothelial degeneration +++ Aneurysm +++ A-V shunts Large area capillary closure	
4 – final	Same lesions plus retinitis proliferans	Endothelial degeneration ++++ Aneurysm +++ Generalized capillary closure	

Modified from Cunha-Vaz [4].

In summary, the abnormalities seen in DR can conceptually be split into three categories: findings resulting from structural retinal neurodegeneration (thinning of the innermost retinal layers and multifocal electroretinography [mfERG] abnormalities); findings resulting from leaking microvasculature (hemorrhages, lipid exudates, and retinal edema); and findings resulting from microvascular alterations resulting in ischemia with a subsequent overproduction of vascular growth factors (cotton-wool spots, intraretinal neovascular abnormalities, preretinal neovascularization, fibrous proliferation, and vitreous hemorrhage).

Clinical Classification of DR

The Diabetic Retinopathy Study (DRS) created the modified Airlie House classification system and added more gradations of severity using 7-field retinography [11, 12]. This classification was developed to classify DR progression to proliferative DR. Fundus imaging of the posterior pole of the retina has been accepted as the reference standard to grade DR for decades and relies on a 20–50° field of view for each of the 7 fields. The standardized 7-field images show hemorrhages, MAs, exudates, cotton-wool spots, intraretinal vascular abnormalities and neovascularization, as well as retinal thickening to be recognized, staged, and quantified in terms of size, number and location. ETDRS (Early Treatment Diabetic Retinopathy Study) grading represents the morphological picture of DR progression and any new information on classification should be evaluated in the context of this well-established classification/grading.

It is recognized that the duration of diabetes and the level of metabolic control condition the development of DR. However, these risk factors do not explain the great variability that characterizes the evolution and rate of progression of the retinopathy in different diabetic individuals.

There is clearly great individual variation in the presentation and course of DR. Many diabetic patients never develop sight-threatening retinal changes after many years of disease, maintaining good visual acuity. However, there are other patients that even after only a few years of diabetes show a retinopathy that progresses rapidly and may not even respond to available treatments. The wide range of retinal changes between different individuals with similar disease duration and metabolic control is well demonstrated in the studies calculating MA turnover. MA values have been shown to have a wide range even in eyes in the same ETDRS retinopathy grade [13] confirming previous observations by Sharp et al. [14] indicating that MA turnover values may represent different microvascular disease activity in different eyes.

If DR is a multifactorial disease in the sense that different factors or different pathways may predominate in different subjects with DR, then it is important that these differences are recognized and possible different phenotypes identified [15].

Our group has proposed three phenotypes of mild nonproliferative DR (NPDR) with different risks for development of vision-threatening complications. Phenotype A, characterized by slow progression, phenotype B, showing predominance of edema and identified as "leaky" phenotype, and phenotype C characterized by increased rates of MA turnover, i.e. increased rates of MA formation and disappearance.

The results of a pooled analysis of four different longitudinal, observational studies of mild NPDR in diabetes type 2 confirmed a series of previous studies distinguishing three different DR phenotypes of disease progression to macular edema, the most frequent vision-threatening complication of DR [16, 17]. This pooled analysis of 882 patients with mild NPDR, ETDRS grades 20–35, enabled the collection of 103 progression events, a number sufficiently high to allow the application of parametric statistics, an objective difficult to achieve considering the slow rate of DR

progression and consequent low number of events [17].

It is noteworthy that this pooled analysis was based on four different studies involving mild NPDR eyes but having the same inclusion criteria, using the same methodology, and having the image analysis performed by the same reading center.

Using only noninvasive procedures, easy to repeat in the clinical practice, the study showed that characterization of mild NPDR phenotypes has a prognostic value. The chance of developing macular edema within 2 years is 7–25 times higher if the patients have increased central retinal thickness (CRT) (phenotype B) and 14–62 times higher if the patients have increased CRT measurements and MA turnover greater or equal to six in a period of 6 months (phenotype C), when comparing with phenotype A patients.

Of great relevance is the finding that phenotype A, characterized by low MA turnover and no signs of increased retinal thickness, representing approximately 50% of the mild NPDR patient population, shows a negative predictive value of 97% for the development of macular edema. This observation has important implications for the management of DR, indicating that a large proportion of eyes presenting initial stages of retinal vascular disease will progress very slowly, and those eyes are not likely to develop macular edema for a period of at least 2 years.

The reason why only a few patients develop retinal disease and progress to vision loss is the crucial question that needs to be answered in order to fully understand the disease evolution.

Multimodal Imaging of Diabetic Retinal Disease

We have now new ways of examining the diabetic retina. With the advent of spectral-domain optical coherence tomography (SD-OCT) and OCT angiography (OCTA), we may for the first time look at the different components of diabetic retinal damage: retinal neurodegeneration, edema, and microvascular changes in a multimodal approach and noninvasively allowing repeated examinations and longitudinal studies to characterize the evolution of retinopathy.

OCT has become the standard clinical imaging tool in retinal disease. In the neuroretina, differences in the density of optical interfaces, which are displayed as intensities in typical OCT images, correspond to the transitions between tissues in the retina as seen on histology. OCT enables a detailed view of the various retinal layers in vivo, and is now the clinical standard for the reliable and repeatable quantification of retinal thickness, significantly enhancing our ability to diagnose and treat DME.

OCTA is a technique that allows in vivo imaging of the retinal capillary bed in a patient-friendly manner without contrast dye [18]. Recent studies done by our group confirmed that retinal neurodegeneration may precede the microvasculopathy of DR and that retinal neurodegeneration may occur in the absence of any signal of microvascular damage [7].

Another recent study done by our group [19] evaluated the changes occurring in 40 eyes in the initial stage of diabetic retinal disease using a combined approach. The OCTA was used to identify and quantify the microvascular alterations. The structural OCT was used to identify and quantify retinal edema, represented by increases in retinal thickness in the full retina and/or in specific layers of the retina, and to identify and quantify the retinal neurodegeneration represented by thinning (decreases vs. normal values) of the innermost retinal layers (nerve fiber and ganglion cell layers) [18, 20].

For microvascular changes, the performance of several features was studied to discriminate the evolution of DR pathology. Features related to microvascular changes such as decreased vessel density in the superficial retina plexus (SRP) and deep retinal plexus (DRP), enlargement of the foveal avascular zone (FAZ) area, and MA turnover were used. Vessel density [18] in the SRP and in the DRP was computed using the software developed by Carl Zeiss Meditec for the Cirrus Angioplex (Fig. 1).

The metrics of vessel density show changes since grades 10–20 in diabetic eyes, but these changes are, in general, not more than 1 SD when compared to the healthy control population. They were more easily detected in the ETDRS inner ring (perifovea) than in the central subfield, and they appear to indicate mild capillary closure (Fig. 2). These changes increase with increased severity of the retinopathy and, therefore, demonstrate well the progression of the retinal microvascular changes. The superficial capillary plexus appeared in this study to show changes earlier, but this finding may be due to the lower standard deviations associated with presently available measurements of the superficial capillary plexus in comparison with the deep capillary plexus. Decreases in vessel density in the SRP correlate well with MA turnover which has been shown to correlate with retinopathy severity [17, 21].

FAZ evaluations followed closely the findings in vessel density, but only measurements of FAZ circularity appeared to have some value in these initial retinopathy stages.

The presence of neurodegeneration demonstrated by thinning of retinal nerve fiber layer (RNFL) was detected in a relatively large percentage of eyes since grades 10–20 (Fig. 3), but does not appear to increase in parallel with retinopathy ETDRS severity. Furthermore, it was not associated with presence or absence of decreased vessel density.

The presence of retinal edema well demonstrated by increased retinal thickness, mainly located initially in the inner nuclear layer (INL) of the retina (Fig. 4), was also a frequent finding since the earliest retinopathy stages confirming previ-

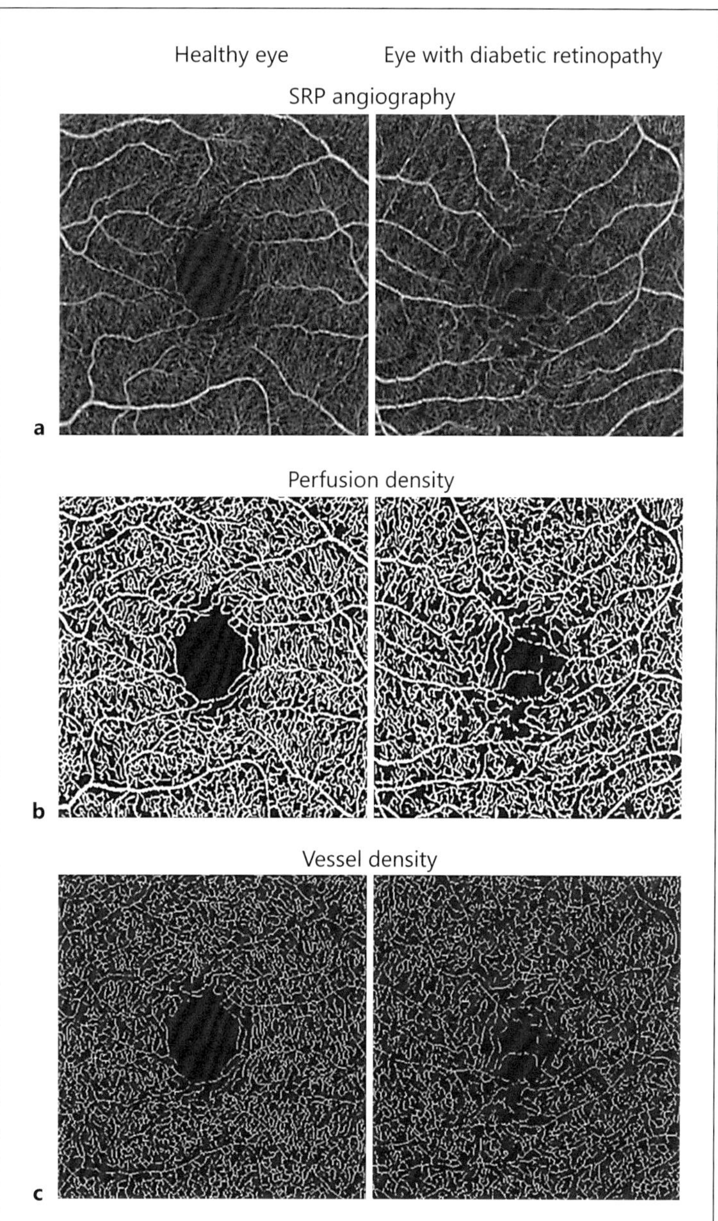

Fig. 1. Image processing steps in microvascular density quantification. Each row shows an example of one aspect of the quantitative measurements for a healthy eye (55-year-old woman) and an eye with diabetic retinopathy (54-year-old man: ETDRS grade 35C; type 2 diabetes for 12 years; hemoglobin 7.2%). **a** Angioplex superficial retinal plexus (SRP) angiography 3 × 3 mm scan. **b** Binarized slab of the SRP image, used for the perfusion density. **c** Skeletonized image used for vessel density. Adapted from Durbin et al. [18].

ous reports [22, 23]. There was also no apparent association between the presence of retinal edema and capillary closure or retinal neurodegeneration. Capillary closure may, indeed, contribute to the relative decrease in the occurrence of retinal edema in the more advanced ETDRS grades.

Looking at the different ETDRS retinopathy severity stages, our findings showed that at levels 10–20, 72.7% of the eyes presented signs of subclinical edema and that 63.6% of eyes showed evidence of some degree of retinal neurodegeneration, when accepting changes of 1 SD from

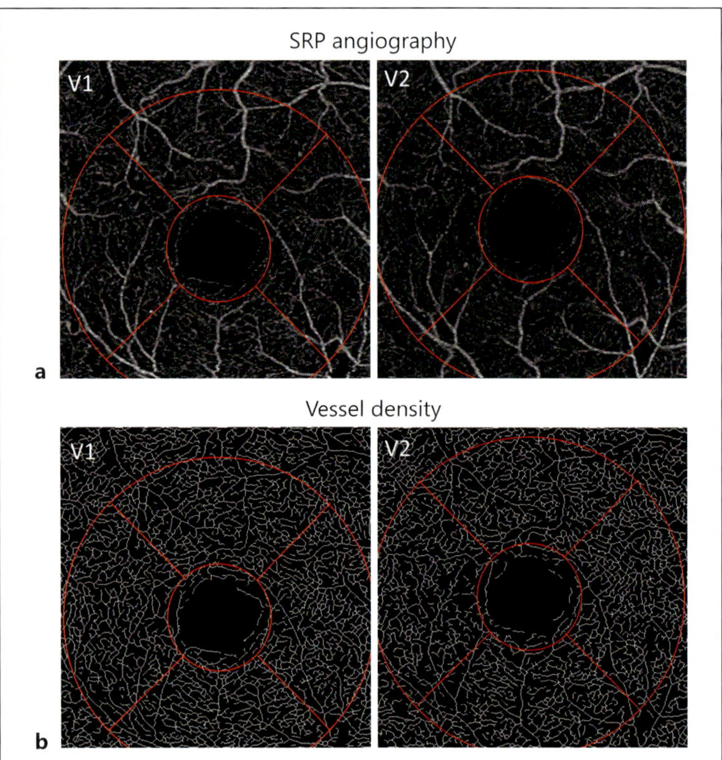

Fig. 2. Right eye with capillarity closure, i.e. decreased vessel density. **a** Slab of the superficial retinal plexus acquired with the angiography 3 × 3 mm protocol from the Zeiss Cirrus AngioPlex. **b** Skeletonized image used for the vessel density. V1 and V2 correspond to the first and second visit. In the first visit, the decrease in the superficial retinal plexus in the inner ring temporal was below 1 SD and in the second visit below 2 SD.

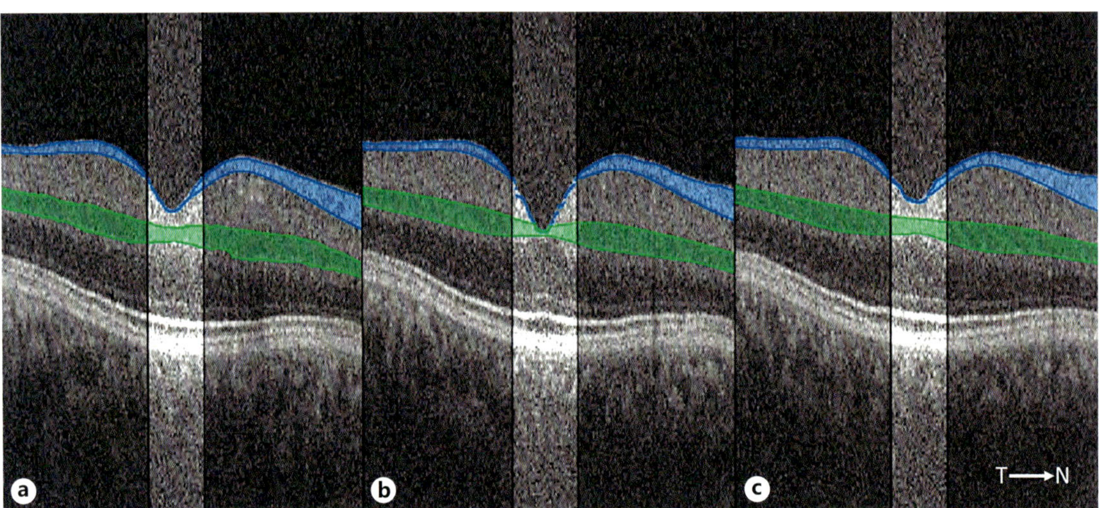

Fig. 3. Right eye with neurodegeneration i.e., thinning of RNFL. Three B-scans of the structural OCT, acquired with the angiography 6 × 6 mm protocol from the Zeiss Cirrus AngioPlex, of an eye with a decreased thickness of the RNFL (1 SD). Image **b** corresponds to the scan acquired at the fovea, and images **a** and **c** at +250 and −250 μm from the fovea, respectively, measured from the inferior to the superior direction. The blue highlighted layer corresponds to the RNFL layer and the green corresponds to the INL layer. The darker areas correspond to the regions outside the central subfield.

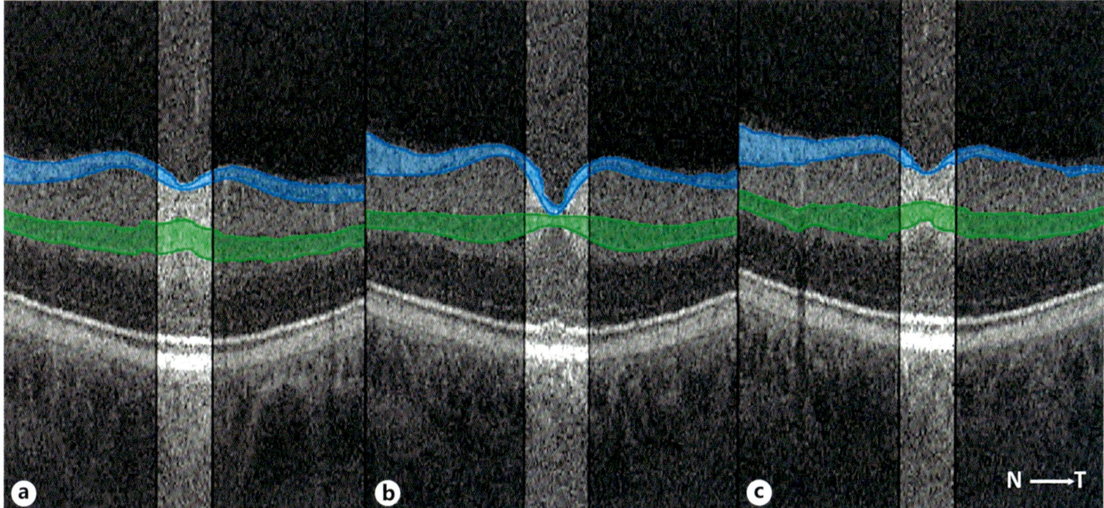

Fig. 4. Left eye with edema. Three B-scans of the structural OCT, acquired with the angiography 6 × 6 mm protocol from the Zeiss Cirrus AngioPlex, of an eye with an increased thickness of the INL (2 SD). Image **b** corresponds to the scan acquired at the fovea, and images **a** and **c** at +250 and −250 μm from the fovea, respectively, measured from the inferior to the superior direction. The blue highlighted layer corresponds to the RNFL layer and the green layer corresponds to the INL layer. The darker areas correspond to the regions outside the central subfield.

the normal population values. The overlap between eyes with the two changes was only 36.4%. Both these changes were better identified in the CSF, again supporting the concept that diabetic retinal disease is initiated in the posterior pole.

Eyes with ETDRS grade level 35 showed the same wide range of changes. Different eyes with the same retinopathy grade showed changes whereas others did not. The presence of edema and retinal neurodegeneration remained at similar levels. However in this ETDRS grade, the retinal thinning may be masked in some eyes by the accumulation of fluid and thickening of the entire retina [24]. Retinal edema is frequent in this retinopathy grade. Decreases in vessel density are now apparent in both SRP and DRP, but these changes are more easily detected in the SRP, reaching now approximately 35.0% of the eyes (2 SD).

Finally, at levels 43–47, decreases in vessel density in the SRP were registered in almost half of the eyes, demonstrating the generalized occurrence of capillary closure at this level.

Our analysis of the initial stages of diabetic retinal disease shows the presence of retinal neurodegeneration, but it does not increase with increased ETDRS severity. It appears to occur independently of the microvascular changes, although it may still have a role as a trigger to the microvascular pathology [25].

Edema was a frequent finding (more than 50% of eyes) since the initial stages being located mainly in the INL, suggesting an alteration of the blood-retinal barrier in the DRP [24]. This observation done in this study may be highly relevant, capable of predicting the eyes that will develop macular edema [13, 22, 23, 26]. The definite evidence of capillary closure, with the metrics available, was registered in both SRP and DRP but was detected earlier in the SRP.

The main conclusion of this study was that the variables that represent microvascular changes (vessel density of SRP and DRP, FAZ area, and

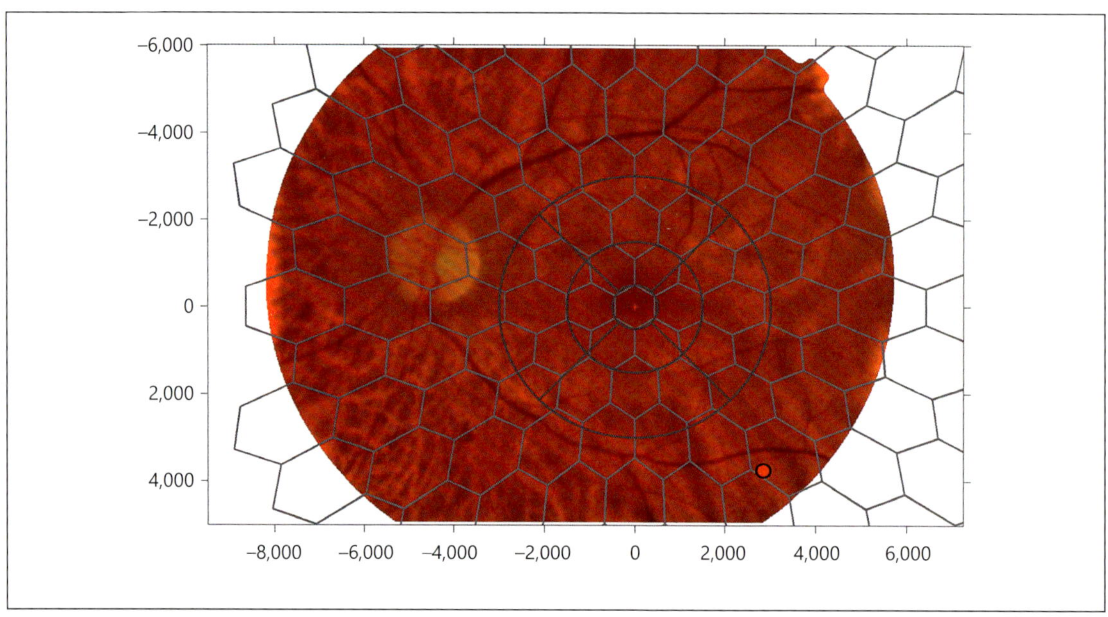

Fig. 5. Multimodal image presenting the functional measurement using mfERG (hexagons grid), the retinal thickness measured using SD-OCT (nine ETDRS grid), and the microaneurysms detected in the CFP (red circle). Example of a case without significant alterations in the mfERG or thickness. A microaneurysm was detected outside the ETDRS grid.

circularity and MA turnover), retinal neurodegeneration (thinning of the RNFL and ganglion cell layer [GCL] + inner plexiform [IPL] layers), and retinal edema (increased thickness of the INL and outer plexiform layer of the retina) show a wide range of values between different eyes in each NPDR ETDRS level, demonstrating that there are very different degrees of microvascular damage, neurodegenerative changes and edema in different eyes in the same retinopathy grade. This conclusion supports the concept of three major phenotypes of retinal disease in diabetes type 2.

Multimodal Analysis of DR Combining Functional and Structural Examinations

Recently, there have been a number of reports suggesting that abnormalities in retinal function can be detected in patients in absence of microvascular abnormalities [27, 28]. In addition, it has been suggested that diabetes-induced retinal neurodysfunction might contribute to the development of retinal microvascular changes [28]. Using either functional measurements such as mfERG or structural assessments such as by SD-OCT, clinical studies have documented the presence of neurodegeneration even before microvascular disease [29, 30].

Neuronal integrity is essential for vision. In the early stages of diabetes, a number of patients presented deficits that they are commonly unaware of in daily life. These deficits included decreased hue discrimination and contrast sensitivity, delayed dark adaptation, visual field changes, and impairment of vision-related quality of life with specific reference to color and peripheral vision [31–33].

A large clinical trial (EUROCONDOR Study) was implemented to evaluate the effects of topically administered neuroprotective agents in di-

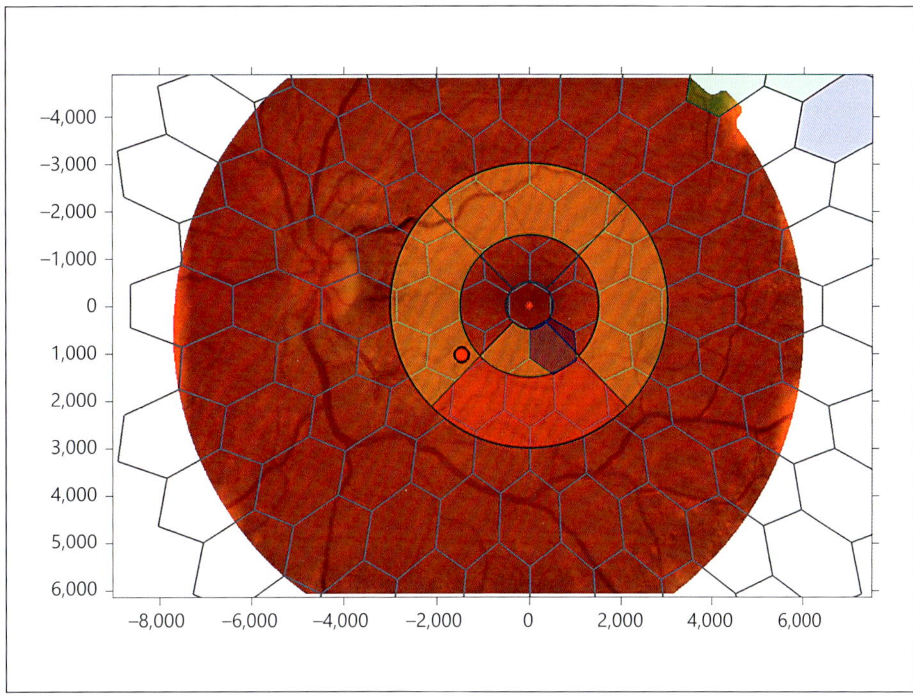

Fig. 6. Multimodal image presenting the functional measurement using mfERG (hexagons grid), the retinal thickness measured using SD-OCT (nine ETDRS grid), and the microaneurysms detected in the CFP (red circle). Example of a case with retinal thickness increases in the outer ring and inner ring inferior quadrant, with microaneurysm detected inside the ETDRS grid and abnormal mfERG response outside the region of interest. The ETDRS area in red and yellow correspond to over 99 and 95%, respectively, of Cirrus HD-OCT retinal thickness normative database. The mfERG hexagons in blue and in light green correspond to implicit time Z-score ≥ 2 and the amplitude Z-score ≤ -2, respectively.

abetic patients with no or mild DR. The trial included 449 patients, aged 45–75 years, with a diagnosis of type 2 diabetes with a duration of >5 years, and an ETDRS level <20 (MA absent) or 20–35 [34].

Taking into account the uniformized criteria chosen for the study, only 58% of diabetic patients with ETDRS <20 (no visible microvascular lesions) showed mfERG abnormalities at baseline (patients with neurodysfunction), while 66% of diabetic patients with ETDRS 20–35 present mfERG abnormalities.

Diabetic patients presented a significantly delayed implicit time, IT (P_1) from rings 3–6 in comparison with an age-matched nondiabetic control group. No influence was found between different ETDRS levels on IT (P_1).

Furthermore, the mean IT of the 6 rings was similar in type 2 diabetic patients with ETDRS <20 or ETDRS level 20–35 (36.66 ± 1.76 vs. 36 ± 1.76).

The mean values of amplitude (P_1) were significantly lower in diabetic patients than in the control group in all rings, with the differences being slightly higher in patients with ETDRS levels 20–35 than in patients without microangiopathic abnormalities. Age was correlated with IT but no relationship was found between

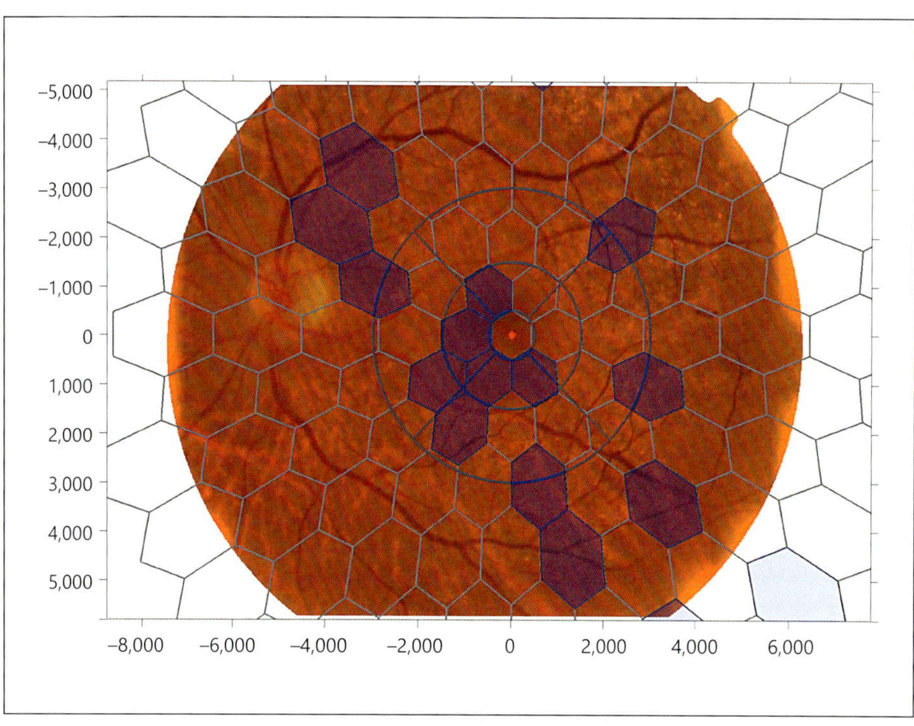

Fig. 7. Multimodal image presenting the functional measurement using mfERG (hexagons grid) and the retinal thickness measured using SD-OCT (nine ETDRS grid). Example of a case with abnormal mfERG response. The mfERG hexagon in blue corresponds to implicit time Z-score ≥ 2.

IT or amplitude with diabetes duration or HbA_{1c} levels.

The average GCL-IPL thickness was significantly lower in eyes of patients with diabetes when compared to the normal population (79.4 ± 7.3 vs. 82.1 ± 6.2 μm; $p < 0.001$); but there was no difference among patients with different ETDRS levels (78.6 ± 7.3 vs. 79.7 ± 7.7; $p = 0.13$). Average RNFL at the optic disc presented no significant differences between patients' eyes and the normal population (89.1 ± 9.7 vs. 89.8 ± 8.5 μm; $p = 0.32$). A total of 41 patients with type 2 diabetes (9.1%) presented values of GCL-IPL or RNFL below the normal range.

The baseline data collected from EURO-CONDOR participants showed abnormalities related to neurodegeneration detected by mfERG or SD-OCT in 118 out of 193 (61%) type 2 diabetic patients with no apparent fundus abnormalities (ETDRS level <20). These findings appear to confirm a neurodysfunctional or neurodegenerative phenotype and are in agreement with previous studies [29, 35–37] supporting the concept that functional impairment related to neurodegeneration is an early event in the diabetic retina. However, in 82 of 256 (32%) diabetic patients with early microvascular impairment (ETDRS 20–35), mfERG abnormalities were not found, confirming the presence of a primarily microvascular or a microangiopathic phenotype. Therefore, it seems that in some of these patients, retinal neurodegeneration does not play an essential role in the development of DR, at least when assessed by mfERG. Multimodal analysis of the eyes superimposing the sites of mfERG alterations, presence of abnormally increased retinal thickness, and location of MAs shows that these alterations occur in most cases in the initial stages of the DR, independently and without any apparent association (Fig. 5–7).

The most important structural damage of the retina detected by SD-OCT was thinning of the GCL-IPL and RNFL layers, although in far fewer eyes/patients in comparison with mfERG abnormalities. However, mfERG abnormalities were absent in around 1/3 of patients with ETDRS level <20 in whom GCL-IPL or RNFL thickness was below the normal range.

Our findings show the existence of a significant proportion of patients with a primarily microvascular or microangiopathic phenotype, whereas other eyes of patients without visible microvascular disease (ETDRS <20) presented abnormalities related to neurodegeneration assessed by either mfERG or SD-OCT, suggesting a neurodysfunctional or neurodegenerative phenotype.

A Novel Classification of DR Based on Multimodal Image Analysis

Vision loss in DR is associated with the occurrence of macular edema or the complications resulting from proliferative DR. The different phenotypic characteristics identify eyes with different risks for disease progression and vision loss. We hereby propose that the identification of the relative role of the three mechanisms of disease (neurodegeneration, edema, and capillary closure) in an eye of a diabetic patient should be the basis of a novel classification of DR (Table 2).

Neurodegeneration identified by OCT-structural analysis (at least 1 SD below normal values) or functional testing can be classified as absent, possible, or definite. In the case of edema, identi-fied using OCT-structural analysis, can be classified as absent, possible (subclinical macula edema) or definite (central involving macular edema). Finally, capillary closure identified by OCTA may also be classified as absent, possible (1 SD below normal value of vessel density in the SCP), or definite (2 SD below normal values of vessel density in SCP).

The relative relevance of these three main mechanisms of the diabetic disease may be explored offering a better characterization of the retinopathy progression and risk of sight-threatening complications, helping clinicians in the management of DR.

Table 2. Categorization of the eye according to mechanisms of the disease

No.	Neurodegeneration	Edema	Capillary closure
0	Absent	Absent	Absent
1	Absent	Possible	Absent
2	Possible	Absent	Absent
3	Possible	Possible	Absent
4	Possible	Definite	Absent
5	Definite	Absent	Absent
6	Definite	Possible	Absent
7	Definite	Definite	Absent
8	Absent	Definite	Absent
9	Absent	Absent	Possible
10	Absent	Possible	Possible
11	Absent	Definite	Possible
12	Possible	Absent	Possible
13	Possible	Possible	Possible
14	Possible	Definite	Possible
15	Definite	Absent	Possible
16	Definite	Possible	Possible
17	Definite	Definite	Possible
18	Absent	Absent	Definite
19	Absent	Possible	Definite
20	Absent	Definite	Definite
21	Possible	Absent	Definite
22	Possible	Possible	Definite
23	Possible	Definite	Definite
24	Definite	Absent	Definite
25	Definite	Possible	Definite
26	Definite	Definite	Definite

References

1 Fong DS, Aiello LP, Ferris FL, Klein R: Diabetic retinopathy. Diabetes Care 2004;27:2540–2553.

2 Yau JWY, Rogers SL, Kawasaki R, et al: Global prevalence and major risk factors of diabetic retinopathy. Diabetes Care 2012;35:556–564.

3 Ashton N: Vascular basement membrane changes in diabetic retinopathy. Montgomery lecture, 1973. Br J Ophthalmol 1974;58:344–366.

4 Cunha-Vaz JG: Pathophysiology of diabetic retinopathy. Br J Ophthalmol 1978; 62:351–355.

5 Cunha-Vaz J, Faria de Abreu JR, Campos AJ: Early breakdown of the blood-retinal barrier in diabetes. Br J Ophthalmol 1975;59:649–656.

6 Waltman SR, Oestrich C, Krupin T, Hanish S, Ratzan S, Santiago J, Kilo C: Quantitative vitreous fluorophotometry. A sensitive technique for measuring early breakdown of the blood-retinal barrier in young diabetic patients. Diabetes 1978;27:85–87.

7 Antonetti DA, Klein R, Gardner TW: Diabetic retinopathy. N Engl J Med 2012;366:1227–1239.

8 Ludovico J, Bernardes R, Pires I, Figueira J, Lobo C, Cunha-Vaz J: Alterations of retinal capillary blood flow in preclinical retinopathy in subjects with type 2 diabetes. Graefe's Arch Clin Exp Ophthalmol 2003;241:181–186.

9 Wong K: Defining Diabetic Retinopathy Severity; in Browning D (eds): Diabetic Retinopathy. New York, Springer, 2010, pp 105–120.

10 Kempen JH, O'Colmain BJ, Leske MC, Haffner SM, Klein R, Moss SE, Taylor HR, Hamman RF: The prevalence of diabetic retinopathy among adults in the United States. Arch Ophthalmol 2004; 122:552–563.

11 Grading diabetic retinopathy from stereoscopic color fundus photographs – an extension of the modified Airlie House classification. ETDRS report number 10. Early Treatment Diabetic Retinopathy Study Research Group. Ophthalmology 1991;98:786–806.

12 Goldberg MF, Jampol LM: Knowledge of diabetic retinopathy before and 18 years after the Airlie House Symposium on Treatment of Diabetic Retinopathy. Ophthalmology 1987;94:741–746.

13 Ribeiro ML, Nunes SG, Cunha-Vaz JG: Microaneurysm turnover at the macula predicts risk of development of clinically significant macular edema in persons with mild nonproliferative diabetic retinopathy. Diabetes Care 2013;36:1254–1259.

14 Sharp PF, Olson J, Strachan F, Hipwell J, Ludbrook A, O'Donnell M, Wallace S, Goatman K, Grant A, Waugh N, McHardy K, Forrester JV: The value of digital imaging in diabetic retinopathy. Health Technol Assess 2003;7:1–119.

15 Grange JD: Retinopathie Diabétique: Rapport à la Societé Française d'Ophthalmologie. Paris, Masson, 1995.

16 Cunha-Vaz J: Phenotypes and biomarkers of diabetic retinopathy. Personalized medicine for diabetic retinopathy: The Weisenfeld Award. Invest Opthalmol Vis Sci 2014;55:5412.

17 Cunha-Vaz J, Ribeiro L, Costa M, Simó R: Diabetic retinopathy phenotypes of progression to macular edema: pooled analysis from independent longitudinal studies of up to 2 years' duration. Invest Opthalmol Vis Sci 2017;58:BIO206.

18 Durbin MK, An L, Shemonski ND, Soares M, Santos T, Lopes M, Neves C, Cunha-Vaz J: Quantification of retinal microvascular density in optical coherence tomographic angiography images in diabetic retinopathy. JAMA Ophthalmol 2017;135:370.

19 Durbin M, Marques I, Mendes L, Torcato S, Catarina N, Santos A, Dalila A, Cunha-Vaz J: Characterization of the initial stages of diabetic retinal disease using optical coherence tomography (OCT) and OCT angiography (OCTA). To be presented at 2018 annual meeting of the ARVO (Association for the Research in Vision and Ophthalmology), Honolulu, Hawaii.

20 Wang RK, An L, Francis P, Wilson DJ: Depth-resolved imaging of capillary networks in retina and choroid using ultrahigh sensitive optical microangiography. Opt Lett 2010;35:1467–1469.

21 Ribeiro L, Bandello F, Tejerina AN, et al: Characterization of retinal disease progression in a 1-year longitudinal study of eyes with mild nonproliferative retinopathy in diabetes type 2. Invest Opthalmol Vis Sci 2015;56:5698.

22 Tejerina AN, Vujosevic S, Varano M, et al: One-year progression of diabetic subclinical macular edema in eyes with mild nonproliferative diabetic retinopathy: location of the increase in retinal thickness. Ophthalmic Res 2015;54:118–123.

23 Bressler NM, Miller KM, Beck RW, Bressler SB, Glassman AR, Kitchens JW, Melia M, Schlossman DK: Observational study of subclinical diabetic macular edema. Eye 2012;26:833–840.

24 Bandello F, Tejerina AN, Vujosevic S, et al: Retinal layer location of increased retinal thickness in eyes with subclinical and clinical macular edema in diabetes type 2. Ophthalmic Res 2015;54:112–117.

25 Sohn EH, van Dijk HW, Jiao C, Kok PHB, Jeong W, Demirkaya N, Garmager A, Wit F, Kucukevcilioglu M, van Velthoven MEJ, DeVries JH, Mullins RF, Kuehn MH, Schlingemann RO, Sonka M, Verbraak FD, Abràmoff MD: Retinal neurodegeneration may precede microvascular changes characteristic of diabetic retinopathy in diabetes mellitus. Proc Natl Acad Sci USA 2016; 113:E2655–E2664.

26 Friedman SM, Almukhtar TH, Baker CW, Glassman AR, Elman MJ, Bressler NM, Maker MP, Jampol LM, Melia M; Diabetic Retinopathy Clinical Research Network: Topical nepafenec in eyes with noncentral diabetic macular edema. Retina 2015;35:944–956.

27 Abcouwer SF, Gardner TW: Diabetic retinopathy: loss of neuroretinal adaptation to the diabetic metabolic environment. Ann NY Acad Sci 2014;1311:174–190.

28 Simó R, Hernández C, European Consortium for the Early Treatment of Diabetic Retinopathy (EUROCONDOR). Neurodegeneration in the diabetic eye: new insights and therapeutic perspectives. Trends Endocrinol Metab 2014;25: 23–33.

29 Harrison WW, Bearse MA, Ng JS, Jewell NP, Barez S, Burger D, Schneck ME, Adams AJ: Multifocal electroretinograms predict onset of diabetic retinopathy in adult patients with diabetes. Invest Opthalmol Vis Sci 2011;52:772.

30 Ng JS, Bearse MA, Schneck ME, Barez S, Adams AJ: Local diabetic retinopathy prediction by multifocal ERG delays over 3 years. Invest Ophthalmol Vis Sci 2008;49:1622–1628.

31 Wolff BE, Bearse MA, Schneck ME, Dhamdhere K, Harrison WW, Barez S, Adams AJ, Adams AJ: Color vision and neuroretinal function in diabetes. Doc Ophthalmol 2015;130:131–139.

32 Trento M, Durando O, Lavecchia S, Charrier L, Cavallo F, Costa MA, Hernández C, Simó R, Porta M; EURO-CONDOR trial Investigators: Vision related quality of life in patients with type 2 diabetes in the EUROCONDOR trial. Endocrine 2017;57:83–88.

33 Jackson GR, Barber AJ: Visual dysfunction associated with diabetic retinopathy. Curr Diab Rep 2010;10:380–384.

34 Santos AR, Ribeiro L, Bandello F, et al: Functional and structural findings of neurodegeneration in early stages of diabetic retinopathy: cross-sectional analyses of baseline data of the EURO-CONDOR project. Diabetes 2017;66: 2503–2510.

35 Reis A, Mateus C, Melo P, Figueira J, Cunha-Vaz J, Castelo-Branco M: Neuro-retinal dysfunction with intact blood-retinal barrier and absent vasculopathy in type 1 diabetes. Diabetes 2014;63: 3926–3937.

36 Han Y, Schneck ME, Bearse MA, Barez S, Jacobsen CH, Jewell NP, Adams AJ: Formulation and evaluation of a predictive model to identify the sites of future diabetic retinopathy. Invest Ophthalmol Vis Sci 2004;45:4106–4112.

37 Ng JS, Bearse MA, Schneck ME, Barez S, Adams AJ: Local diabetic retinopathy prediction by multifocal ERG delays over 3 years. Invest Opthalmol Vis Sci 2008;49:1622.

José Cunha-Vaz
AIBILI – Association for Innovation and Biomedical Research on Light and Image
Azinhaga de Santa Comba, Celas
3000-548 Coimbra (Portugal)
E-Mail cunhavaz@aibili.pt

Cunha-Vaz J, Koh A (eds): Imaging Techniques.
ESASO Course Series. Basel, Karger, 2018, vol 10, pp 102–123 (DOI: 10.1159/000489193)

Multimodal Imaging

Federico Corvi[a] · José Cunha-Vaz[b] · Giovanni Staurenghi[a]

[a]Eye Clinic, Department of Biomedical and Clinical Science "Luigi Sacco," Sacco Hospital, University of Milan, Milan, Italy;
[b]Association for Innovation and Biomedical Research on Light and Image (AIBILI), Coimbra, Portugal

Abstract

Multimodal imaging is becoming essential in the modern clinical practice to perform a correct diagnosis. As several diseases can present a similar appearance by the same imaging modality, the use of different imaging tools represents the gold standard strategy for the successful management of retinal disorders. In this chapter, we describe the impact of multimodal imaging approach in the evaluation of age-related macular degeneration.

© 2018 S. Karger AG, Basel

In the modern ophthalmic practice, the use of different imaging modalities is essential and has become the standard of care for successful management of retinal disorders. In fact, it is uncommon to rely on a single imaging modality to determine diagnosis and therapy and when analyzed together, different imaging modalities can increase diagnostic sensitivity and specificity [1]. However, each imaging technique has unique advantages and limitations and requires training for application and interpretation.

In this contest, the term multimodal imaging has been defined as the combination of more than one imaging modality to provide improved clinical assessment, diagnostics, and therapeutic monitoring (Fig. 1) [2].

Color fundus photography is one of the most important imaging techniques, as it replicates the view of the retina by ophthalmoscopy. Color fundus images are easy to read and document findings seen on fundus examination [3]. Color fundus photographs have traditionally been captured using flash-based systems using white light; however, they can be affected by several factors such as media opacities. The recent introduction of LED source with a broad spectrum can change the appearance of fundus features such as melanoma, hemangioma, etc. Also, multicolor images can be generated by confocal scanning laser ophthalmoscopy through the use of multiple lasers of different wavelengths (infrared, red, green, blue lights) resulting in pseudocolor representations [4].

Fundus autofluorescence is another essential imaging technique that provides indirect information regarding retinal pigment epithelium function and physiology [5]. A light at a certain wavelength excites fluorophores of retinal tissue, and the generated light with longer wavelength is ac-

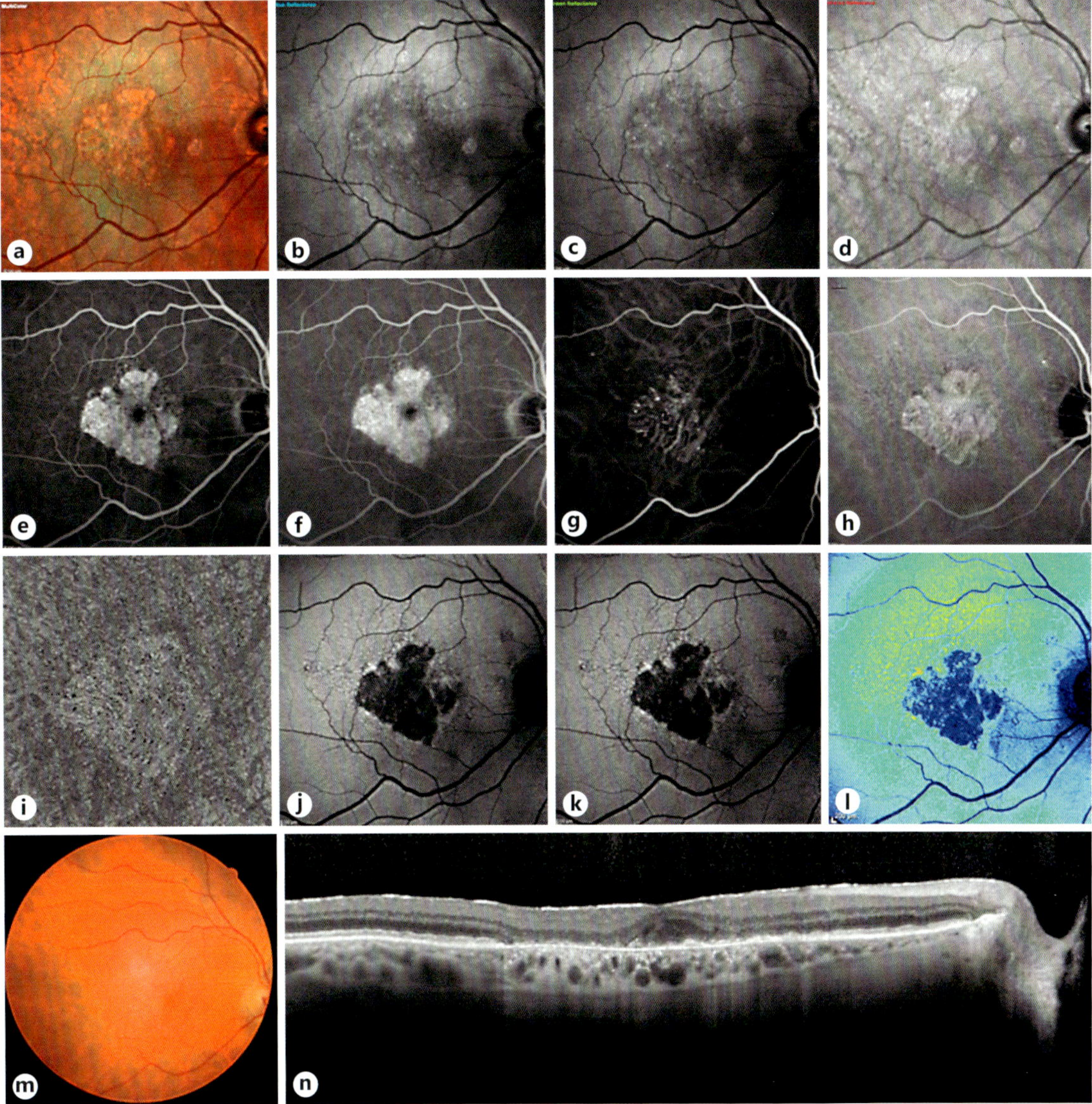

Fig. 1. Multimodal imaging of a patient with geographic atrophy. Multicolor image (**a**), blue reflectance (**b**), green reflectance (**c**), infrared reflectance (**d**), early phase (**e**) and late phase (**f**) of fluorescein angiography, early phase (**g**) and late phase (**h**) of indocyanine green angiography, optical coherence tomography angiography at choriocapillaris segmentation (**i**), blue fundus autofluorescence (**j**), green autofluorescence (**k**), color-coded quantitative fundus autofluorescence (**l**), color fundus photography (**m**), and spectral domain optical coherence tomography (**n**) of geographic atrophy.

quired. The main fluorophores originate with the blue-green light as lipofuscin accumulating in the retinal pigment epithelium [5]. Decreased signal may be observed as a result of lack of excitation light reaching the fluorophores (e.g., blocking from the luteal pigment or vessels or media opacities) or as an indication of loss of the retinal pigment epithelium and photoreceptors. An increased signal may be produced by an excessive accumulation or better visualization due to the lack of retinal tissue of lipofuscin or lipofuscin-like material in or outside retinal pigment epithelium cells (e.g., the surrounding areas of geographic atrophy [GA], vitelliform macular dystrophy, chronic central serous chorioretinopathy) [6, 7].

Fluorescein angiography (FA) and indocyanine green angiography (ICGA) are dynamic examinations used to evaluate the retinal and choroidal vascular circulation. Fluorescein absorbs blue-green light and emits green light, while indocyanine green is imaged by the infrared wavelength. FA and ICGA offer many advantages including dynamic information regarding the transit of blood as well as identification of neovascularization, dye leakage, areas of nonperfusion, and vascular abnormalities [8, 9].

Another important imaging technique is optical coherence tomography (OCT) that has revolutionized the imaging of the retina, becoming a fundamental examination. It produces detailed images with high resolution of the various retinal and choroidal layers providing new insight into several retinal diseases [10].

Recently, OCT angiography (OCTA) has been introduced in the clinical practice offering the opportunity to noninvasively visualize different retinal capillary layers without the need of dye injection [11, 12]. Differently from FA and ICGA, it allows the visualization of 3-dimensional micro-architecture of the vessels. OCTA could be used to perform qualitative and quantitative evaluation of the vascular plexus of the retina adding new insight into the pathogenesis and prognosis of several diseases.

To understand the importance of multimodal imaging approach, we can analyze how the evaluation and classification of age-related macular degeneration (AMD) changed over the time.

In the past, based on FA, neovascularizations were classified only into 2 main patterns: "occult" or "poorly defined" and "classic" or "well-defined" lesions according to their fluorescein angiographic appearance [13]. However, the angiographic distinction between a subretinal and a subpigment ep-

ithelial membrane was not always easy and in some cases impossible. The advent of ICGA facilitated the detection and demarcation of occult or poorly defined neovascularizations in contrast to classic lesions providing more detailed representation of the normal and pathological choroidal vasculature [9]. The use of flash ICGA introduced 2 terms: "plaque" and "hot spot." Also, confocal dynamic ICGA was able to detect the anatomic characteristics of the lesions (e.g., the "racquet-like" and the "umbrella-like" pattern) leading to the discovery of 2 new pathological entities as "polypoidal choroidal vasculopathy" (PCV) and "retinal angiomatous proliferation" [14, 15]. Later, the introduction of OCT offered the opportunity to visualize and recognize different layers of the retina with high resolution adding new useful information [10].

The advent of OCTA offered the opportunity to noninvasively visualize the neovascular networks and correlate the OCTA appearance with the other imaging techniques and observe new findings [16].

Herein, we evaluate several ocular disorders by the multimodal imaging approach.

Type 1 Neovascularization

Type 1 or occult neovascularization is the most common form of neovascularization in AMD, and it occurs beneath the retinal pigment epithelium [13, 17].

FA reveals the neovascular lesion as late leakage of undetermined source, defined as areas of leakage at the level of the retinal pigment epithelium in the late phase of the angiogram without well-demarcated areas of hyperfluorescence discernible in the early phase of the angiogram that account for the leakage, or as fibrovascular pigment epithelial detachment defined as areas of irregular elevation of the retinal pigment epithelium detectable on stereoscopic angiography consisting of an area of stippled hyperfluorescence noted within 1 to 2 min after fluorescein injection

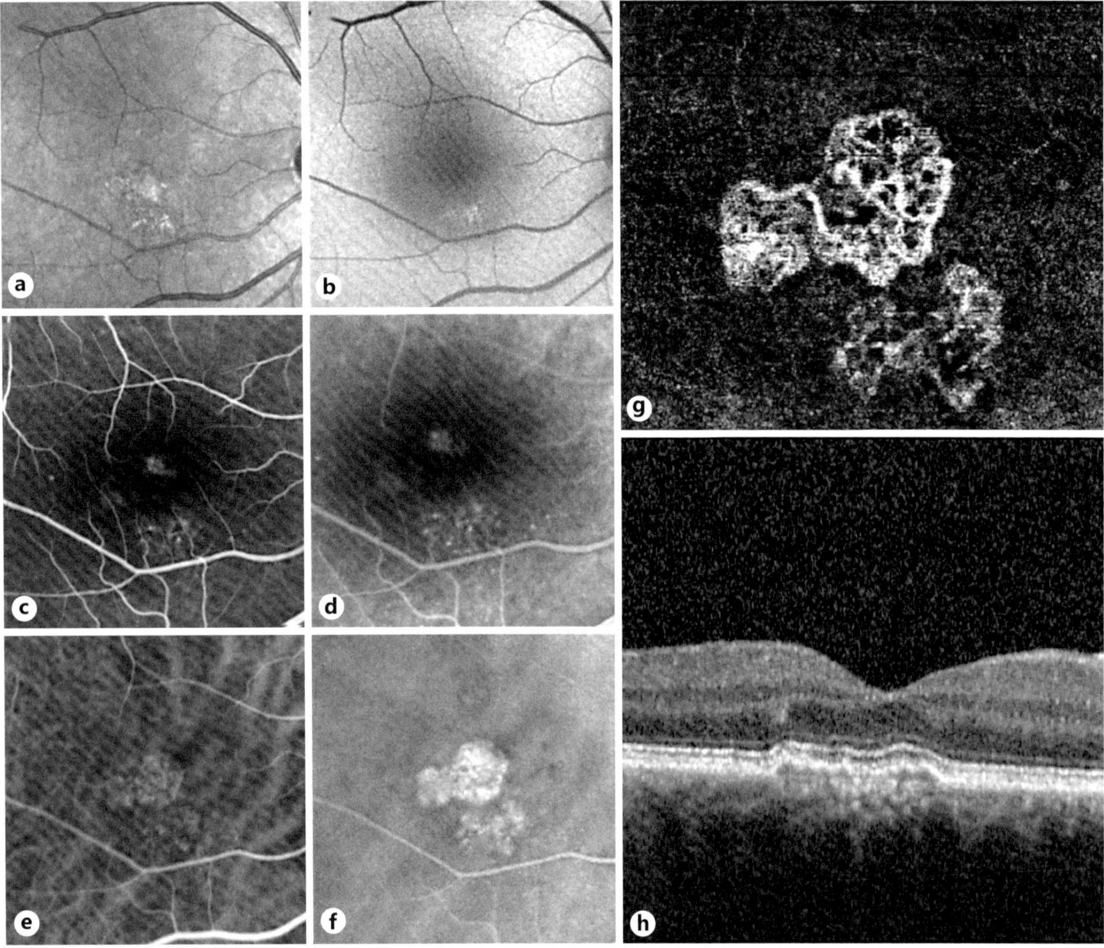

Fig. 2. Multimodal imaging of quiescent type 1 neovascularization. Infrared reflectance (**a**) and fundus autofluorescence (**b**) showing fine alteration of retinal pigment epithelium. Early (**c**) and late phase (**d**) of fluorescein angiography revealing pinpoints of hyperfluorescence. Early (**e**) and late phase (**f**) of indocyanine green angiography showing central hyperfluorescent area corresponding to type 1 neovascularization with similar appearance of optical coherence tomography angiography (**g**). **h** Optical coherence tomography displaying a flat elevation of retinal pigment epithelium with major axis in the horizontal plane.

with leakage within 10 min. However, ICGA could reveal polypoidal or branching neovascular network under these 2 lesions which could respond to treatment in a different way. OCT localized the vessels between the Bruch's membrane and the retinal pigment epithelium as irregularity of retinal pigment epithelium. OCTA reveals the neovascular network with well-defined margins at the choriocapillaris segmentation (Fig. 2, 3).

Type 2 Neovascularization

Type 2 neovascularization is characterized by the growth of the neovascular tissue through the retinal pigment epithelium-Bruch's membrane-choriocapillaris complex to the subretinal space [13]. On FA, these lesions are usually "well-defined" or "classic," as they present a well-demarcated area of hyperfluorescence in the early phase of the

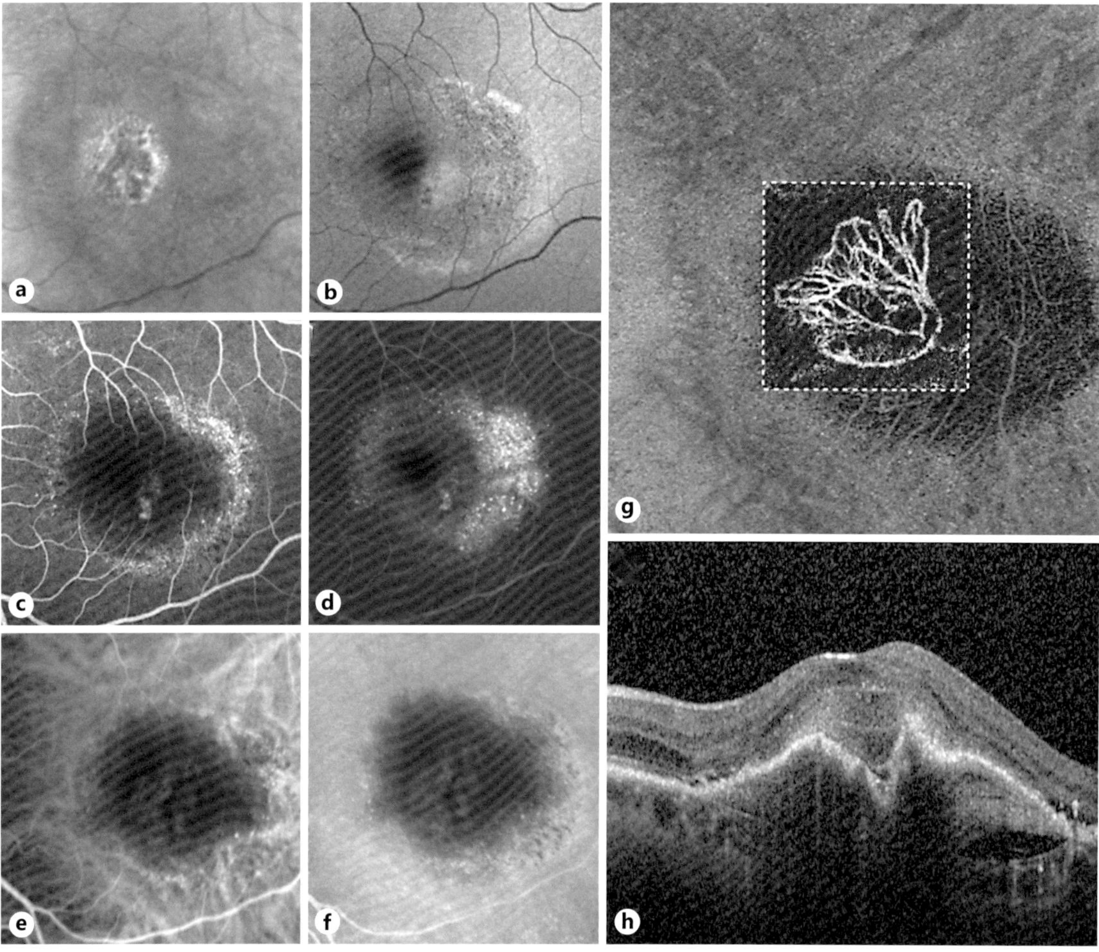

Fig. 3. Multimodal imaging of type 1 neovascularization. Infrared reflectance (**a**) and fundus autofluorescence (**b**) showing abnormalities of retinal pigment epithelium. Early (**c**) and late phase (**d**) of fluorescein angiography revealing pinpoints of hyperfluorescence. Early (**e**) and late phase (**f**) of indocyanine green angiography showing central hyperfluorescent area corresponding to type 1 neovascularization, well visible on optical coherence tomography angiography (**g**). **h** Optical coherence tomography displaying the detachment of retinal pigment epithelium with subretinal fluid and subretinal hyperreflective material.

angiogram, while in the late phase they present a progressive pooling of dye in the overlying subsensory retinal space which usually obscures the boundaries of the choroidal neovascularization (CNV). In the case of type 3 neovascularization, FA sometimes cannot help in the correct identification, while dynamic ICGA reveals in the early phase the neovascular network and helps to identify the lesions.

OCT localizes type 2 neovascularization above the retinal pigment epithelium with disorganization of the overlying inner segment/ outer segment junction and subretinal and intraretinal fluid. However, intraretinal fluid predominates with type 2 lesions rather than subretinal fluid. In larger and older lesions, the neovessels may form a hyperreflective band overlying the retinal pigment epithelium with

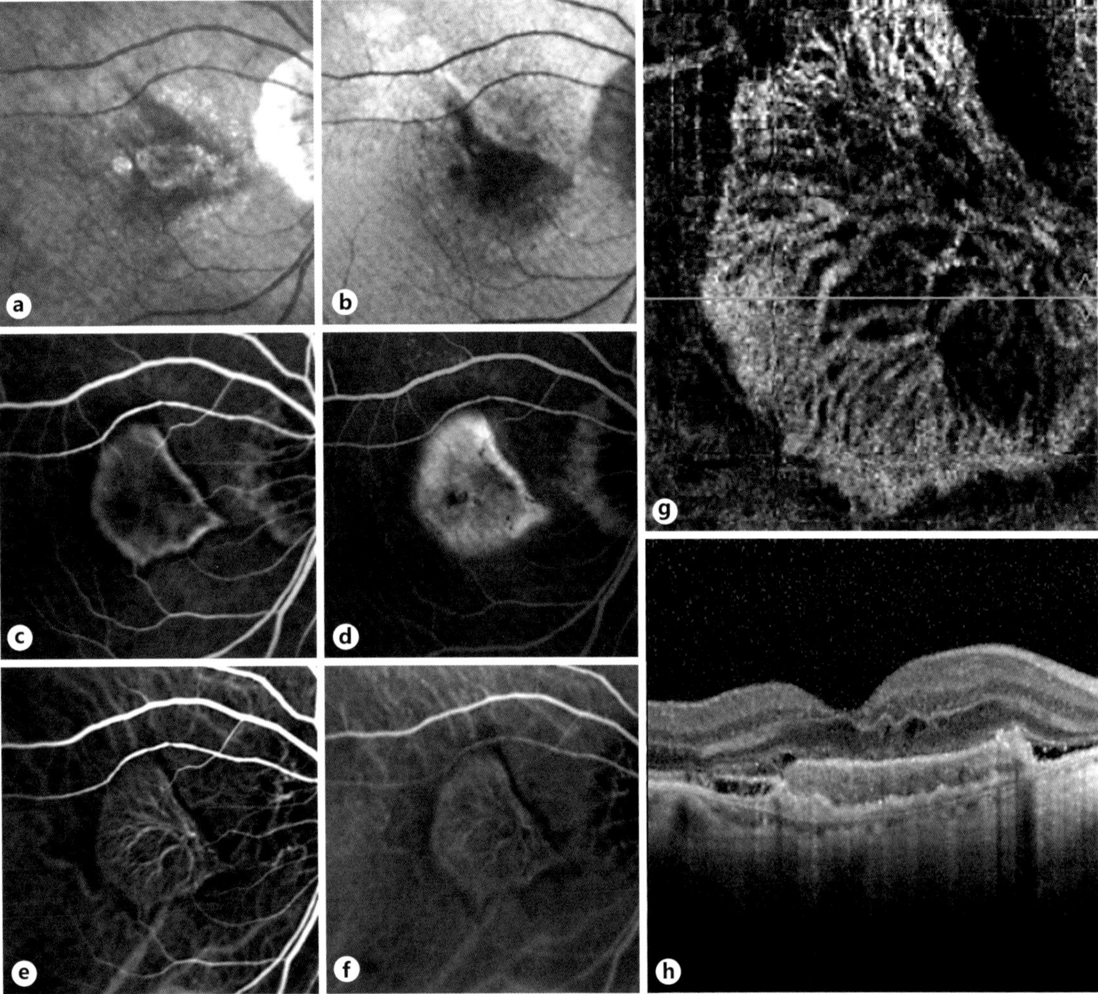

Fig. 4. Multimodal imaging of type 2 neovascularization. Infrared reflectance (**a**) and fundus autofluorescence (**b**) revealing abnormalities of retinal pigment epithelium. Early (**c** and **e**) and late phase (**d** and **f**) of fluorescein angiography and indocyanine green angiography showing a well-defined neovascular network with leakage in the late phases. **g** Optical coherence tomography angiography displaying the neovascular network very similar to indocyanine green angiography appearance and with well-visible and defined margins. **h** Optical coherence tomography showing the neovascularization above the retinal pigment epithelium with disorganization of the overlying inner segment/outer segment junction, subretinal and intraretinal fluid.

substantial thinning and disorganization of the overlying and thinning of the outer nuclear layer (Fig. 4, 5) [18].

However, it is uncommon to find only a type 2 lesion, as type 2 neovascularization is typically connected with type 1. In fact, type 2 neovascularization is common in other disorders where there is an alteration of the retinal pigment epithelium-Bruch's membrane complex to pathological myopia with lacquer cracks (Fig. 6), punctate inner choroidopathy, multifocal choroiditis, angioid streaks (Fig. 7), choroidal rupture (Fig. 8) and idiopathic type 2 neovascularization (Fig. 9).

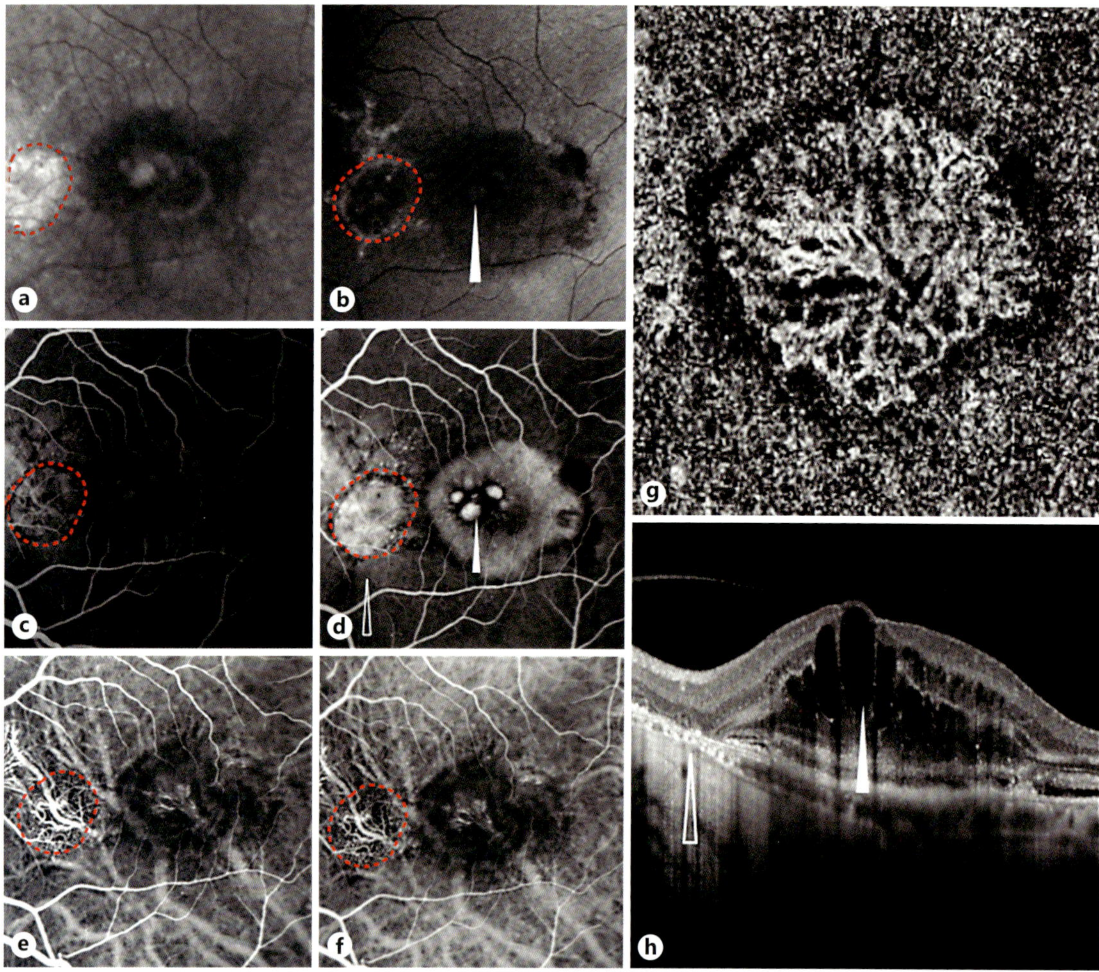

Fig. 5. Multimodal imaging of type 2 neovascularization. Infrared reflectance (**a**) and fundus autofluorescence (**b**) showing a nasal area of atrophy as hyperreflective and hypofluorescent (dotted red circular line), a central hypofluorescent area with small hyperfluorescent points (arrowhead) corresponding to intraretinal fluid. Fluorescein angiography (**c** and **d**) showing a type 2 neovascularization with well-evident leakage and hyperfluorescent cystoid spaces (arrowhead) in the late phase and staining of the dye in the nasal atrophic area. The stereo-indocyanine green angiography (**e** and **f**) and optical coherence tomography angiography (**g**) displaying the neovascular network with well-defined margins. **h** Optical coherence tomography revealing the neovascularization above the retinal pigment epithelium with disorganization of the overlying inner segment/outer segment junction, subretinal fluid and intraretinal cystoid spaces (arrowhead), and nasal hypertransmission of the signal (open arrowhead) corresponding to the atrophic area.

Type 3 Neovascularization

In 1992, Hartnett et al. [19] first described a retinal angiomatous lesion associated with AMD causing retinal pigment epithelium detachment. There has been considerable debate regarding whether this form of neovascularization originates from the retinal circulation (as proposed by Yannuzzi et al. [20]) or the choroidal circulation (as proposed by Gass et al. [21]). Yannuzzi's group proposed a

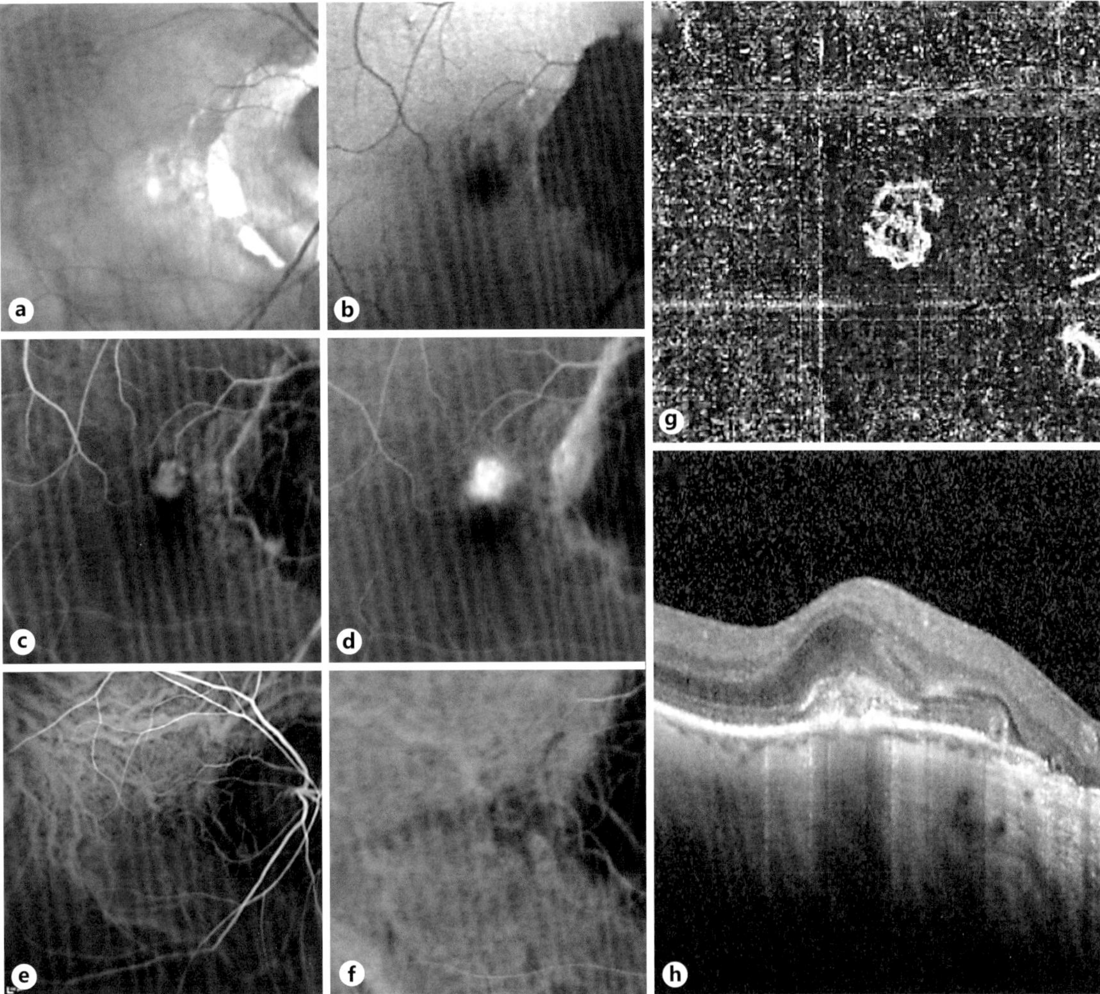

Fig. 6. Multimodal imaging of type 2 neovascularization secondary to pathological myopia. Infrared reflectance (**a**) and blue autofluorescence (**b**) revealing the fundus abnormalities related to pathological myopia. Early phase of fluorescein angiography (**c**) showing the type 2 neovascularization as a hyperfluorescent area that becomes more intense with moderate leakage in the late phase (**d**). Early phase (**e**) and late phase (**f**) of indocyanine green angiography and optical coherence tomography angiography (**g**) revealing the neovascular network with well-circumscribed appearance at the border of atrophy. **h** Optical coherence tomography showing the subretinal hyperreflective material corresponding to the neovascular lesion.

3-stage classification in which stage 1 is characterized by the presence of initial intraretinal neovascularization, in stage 2 the intraretinal neovascularization extends into the subretinal space forming subretinal neovascularization and retinal-retinal anastomosis, and in stage 3 the neovascularization extends deeper forming a retinal-choroidal anastomosis with an underlying vascularized pigment epithelial detachment.

However, the term type 3 neovascularization has been proposed overcoming both hypotheses regarding the origin of this neovascular proliferative process that affects primarily the neurosensory retina [22, 23].

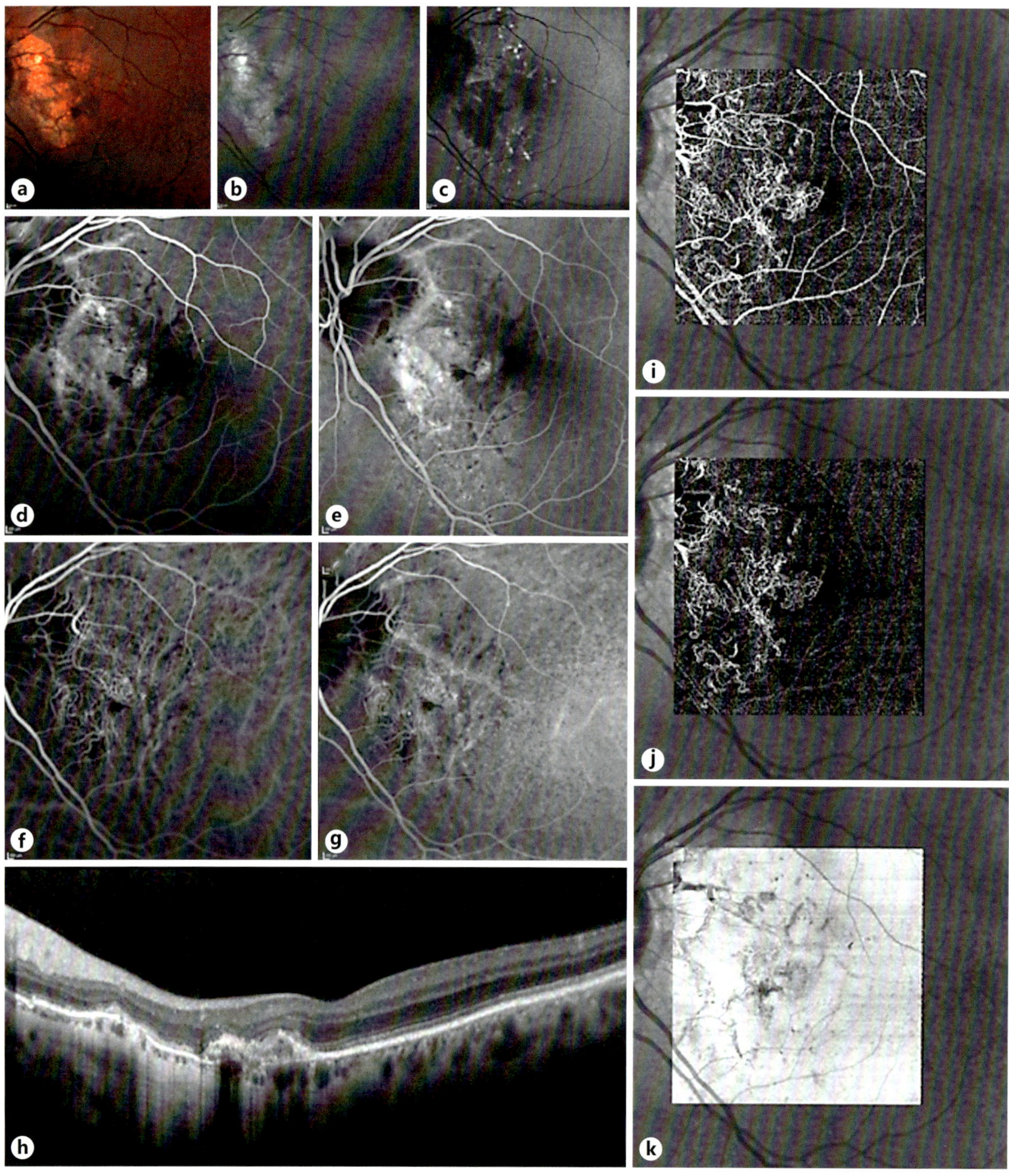

Fig. 7. Multimodal imaging of type 2 neovascularization secondary to angioid streaks. Multicolor imaging (**a**), infrared reflectance (**b**), and blue autofluorescence (**c**) revealing the fundus alterations secondary to angioid streaks. Early phase of fluorescein angiography (**d**) and indocyanine green angiography (**f**) showing a hyperfluorescent area that becomes more intense with moderate leakage in the late phase (**e** and **g**, respectively), as type 2 neovascularization. **h** Optical coherence tomography displaying the area of atrophy with the neovascular tissue above the retinal pigment epithelium without sub-/intraretinal fluid. Optical coherence tomography angiography without projection artifacts (**i**) and with projection artifacts (**j**) showing a choroidal neovascularization with a defined network that closely followed the trajectory of angioid streak, well appreciable on the en-face optical coherence tomography (**k**).

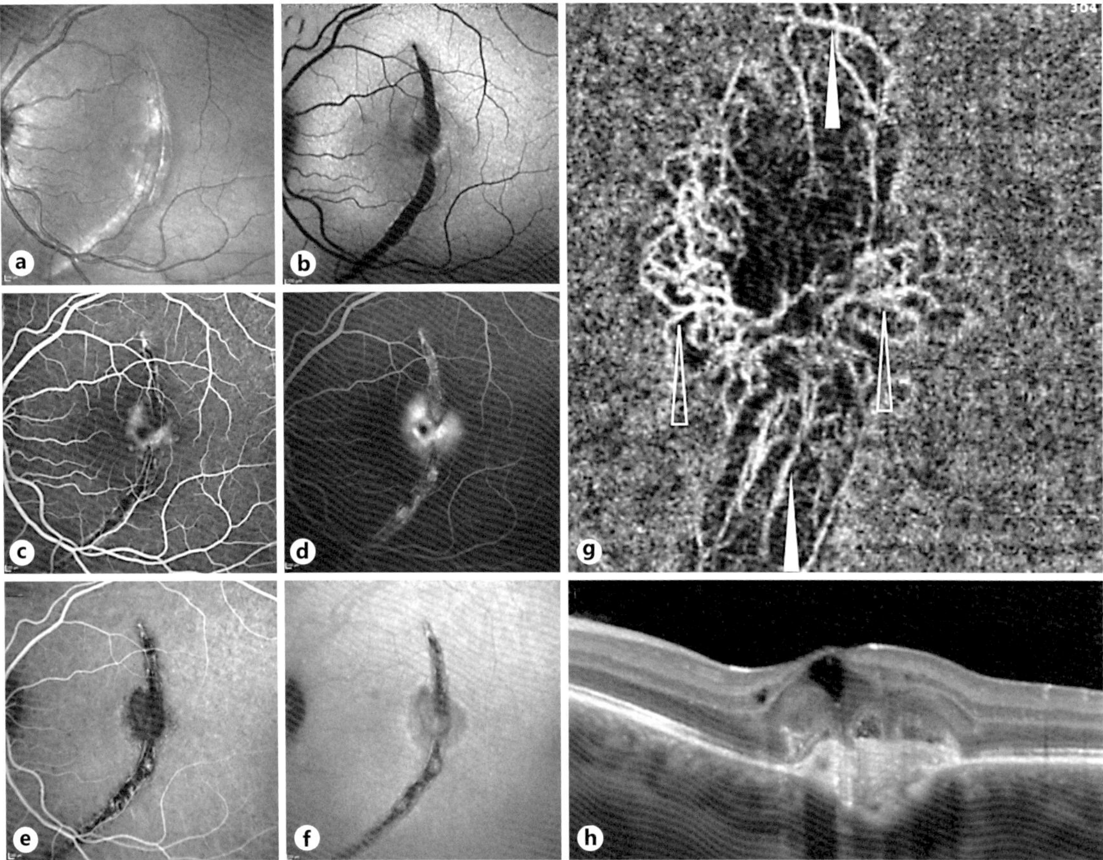

Fig. 8. Multimodal imaging of type 2 neovascularization secondary to choroidal rupture. Infrared reflectance (**a**) and blue autofluorescence (**b**) showing a linear hypofluorescent area surrounded by mild hypofluorescent area. Fluorescein angiography (**c** and **d**) and indocyanine green angiography (**e** and **f**) revealing the choroidal rupture as a hypofluorescent area with a central hyperfluorescence that becomes more intense with moderate leakage in the late phase due to type 2 neovascularization. **g** Optical coherence tomography angiography displaying the choroidal rupture as a regular line of severe choriocapillary rarefaction with projection of superficial retinal vessels (arrowheads) and a well-defined tangled network (open arrowheads). **h** Optical coherence tomography revealing the rupture of retinal pigment epithelium, Bruch's membrane, and choriocapillaris with subretinal hyperreflective material and intraretinal cystoid space.

Multimodal imaging confirmed that the early appearance of type 3 neovascularization is characterized by an intraretinal vascular complex at the deep capillary plexus associated with telangiectatic vessels. Sometimes, intraretinal proliferation seemed to evolve simultaneously with type 1 neovascularization [24]. The origin of this neovascularization may originate from both circulations simultaneously as initial focal retinal prolif-eration and progression or focal retinal proliferation with preexisting or simultaneous choroidal proliferation, or initial focal choroidal proliferation and progression.

As these lesions originate from both the retinal and choroidal circulations, they never originate within the foveal avascular zone but at the near border or a variable distance and from the terminal portions of third-order arterioles and venules [23].

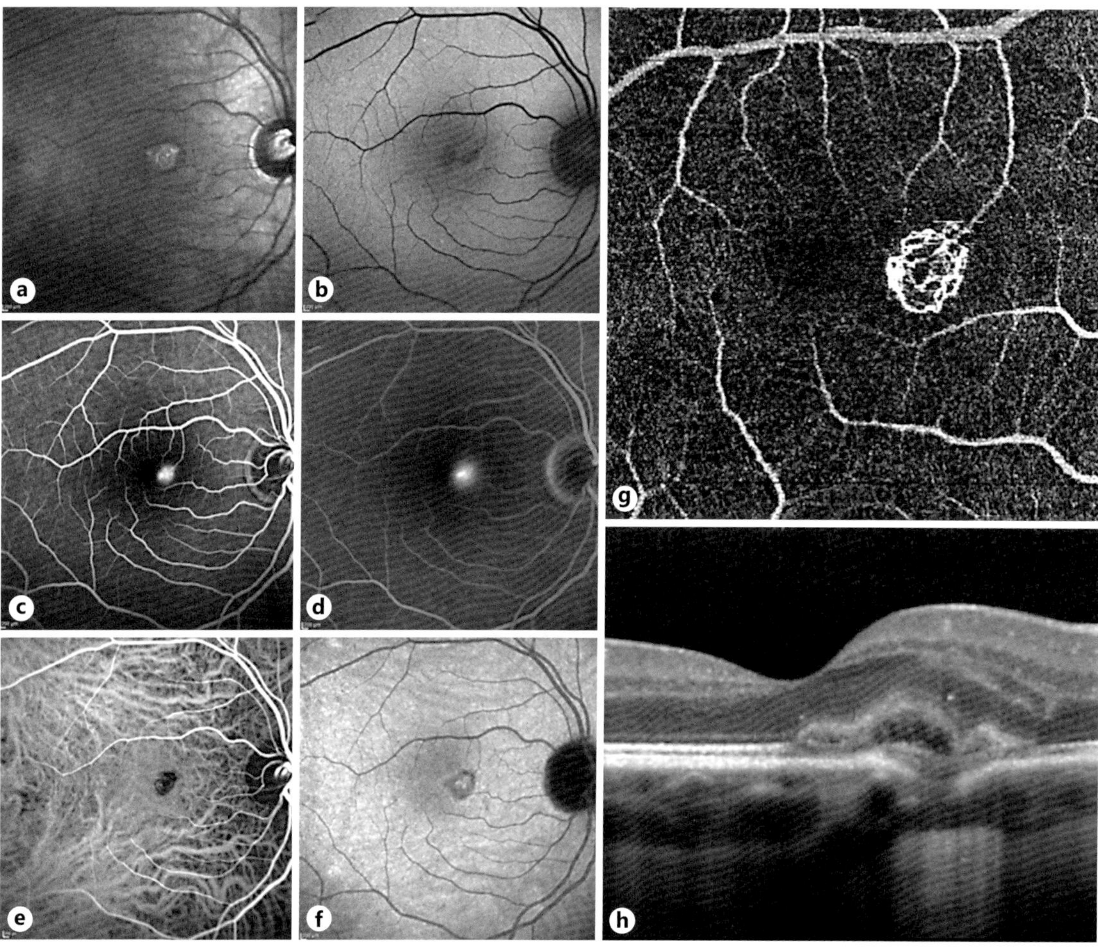

Fig. 9. Multimodal imaging of idiopathic type 2 neovascularization. Infrared reflectance (**a**) and blue autofluorescence (**b**) displaying the central lesion. Early phase (**c**) and late phase (**d**) of fluorescein angiography revealing the type 2 neovascularization as hyperfluorescent with mild leakage. Indocyanine green angiography (**e** and **f**) and optical coherence tomography angiography (**g**) showing the neovascular lesion. **h** Optical coherence tomography displaying the neovascular lesion above the retinal pigment epithelium with subretinal hyperreflective material.

Typically, color fundus photography reveals the presence of small and focal intraretinal hemorrhage. FA and ICGA show type 3 neovascularization as a hyperfluorescent intraretinal vascular complex which appears in the late phase as a leakage area. The leakage in the late phase of ICGA is a unique feature of type 3 CNV. In the case of retinal-retinal anastomosis, stereo images are able to show the connection between the retinal and choroidal vasculature. In the early stage, OCT is usually characterized by intraretinal cyst without neurosensory retinal detachment and retinal pigment epithelium detachment, while in the late stages it reveals the presence of serous retinal pigmented epithelium detachment and retinal pigmented epithelium detachment with retinal-choroidal anastomosis (Fig. 10).

OCTA can be very useful to visualize the neovascular lesion as a discrete high-flow linear structure extending from the middle retinal layers

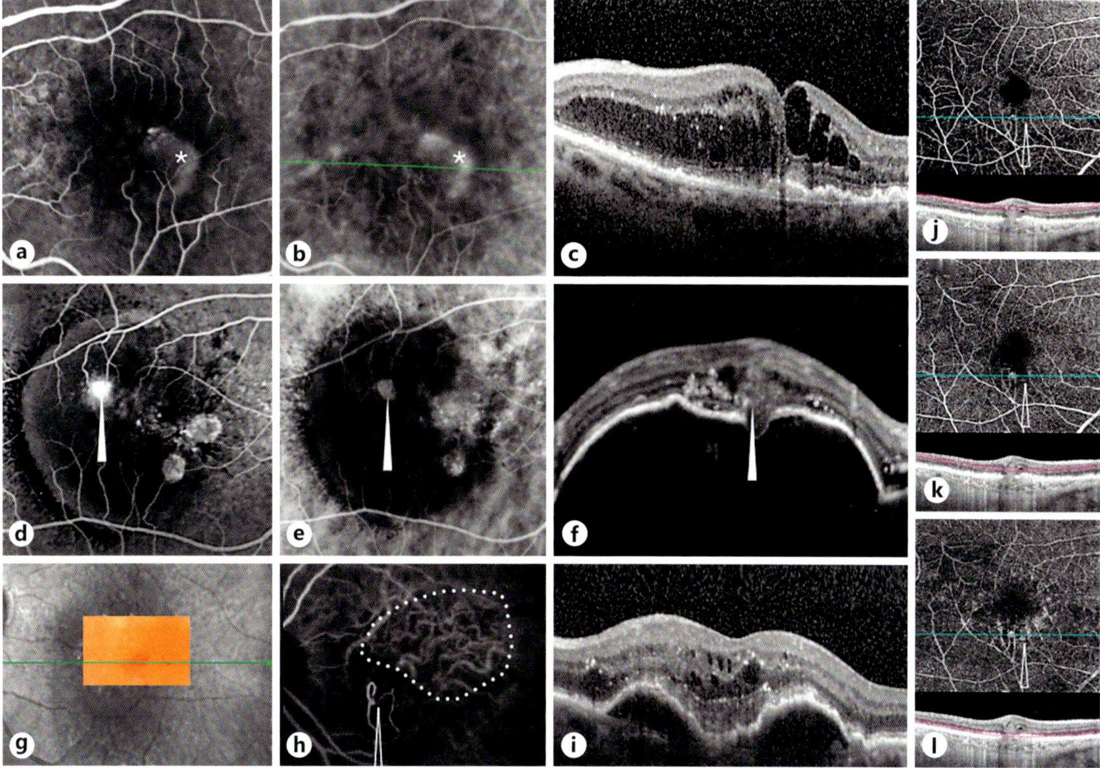

Fig. 10. Multimodal imaging of type 3 neovascularization. Fluorescein angiography (**a**) and indocyanine green angiography (**b**) revealing the neovascularization (asterisks). **c** Optical coherence tomography showing the detachment of retinal pigment epithelium with intraretinal cystoid space. Fluorescein angiography (**d**) and indocyanine green angiography (**e**) displaying large detachment of retinal pigment epithelium as a round hyperfluorescent and hypofluorescent area, respectively, with central hyperfluorescence (arrowheads). **f** Optical coherence tomography showing detachment of retinal pigment epithelium with intraretinal vascular complex emanating from the deep capillary plexus (arrowhead) and underlying defect in the retinal pigment epithelium and intraretinal cystoid space. Color fundus photography (**g**) displaying the hemorrhage, and indocyanine green angiography (**h**) showing the retinal-retinal anastomosis (open arrowhead) with the coexistence of a type 1 neovascularization (dotted circle). **i** Optical coherence tomography revealing detachment of retinal pigment epithelium with intraretinal cystoid space. **j–l** Optical coherence tomography angiography showing a tuft-shaped, high-flow lesion (open arrowheads) in the outer retinal layers abutting into the subretinal pigment epithelium space.

into the deep retina and occasionally also past the retinal pigment epithelium in the presence of deepening neovascular complex.

Polypoidal Choroidal Vasculopathy

Concerning the definition of PCV, there is some controversy as some authors used the term PCV to identify a distinct clinical entity, while other authors used this term to describe a focal morphological manifestation within the neovascular lesions [25]. Type 1 neovascularization is characterized by the presence of pathological vessels under the retinal pigment epithelium [13]. In this context, focal polypoidal changes of the neovascular tissue could be found. The term "polypoidal CNV" would therefore seem appropriate to describe all neovascular complexes that demonstrate polypoidal changes (Fig. 11) [26]. Also, the

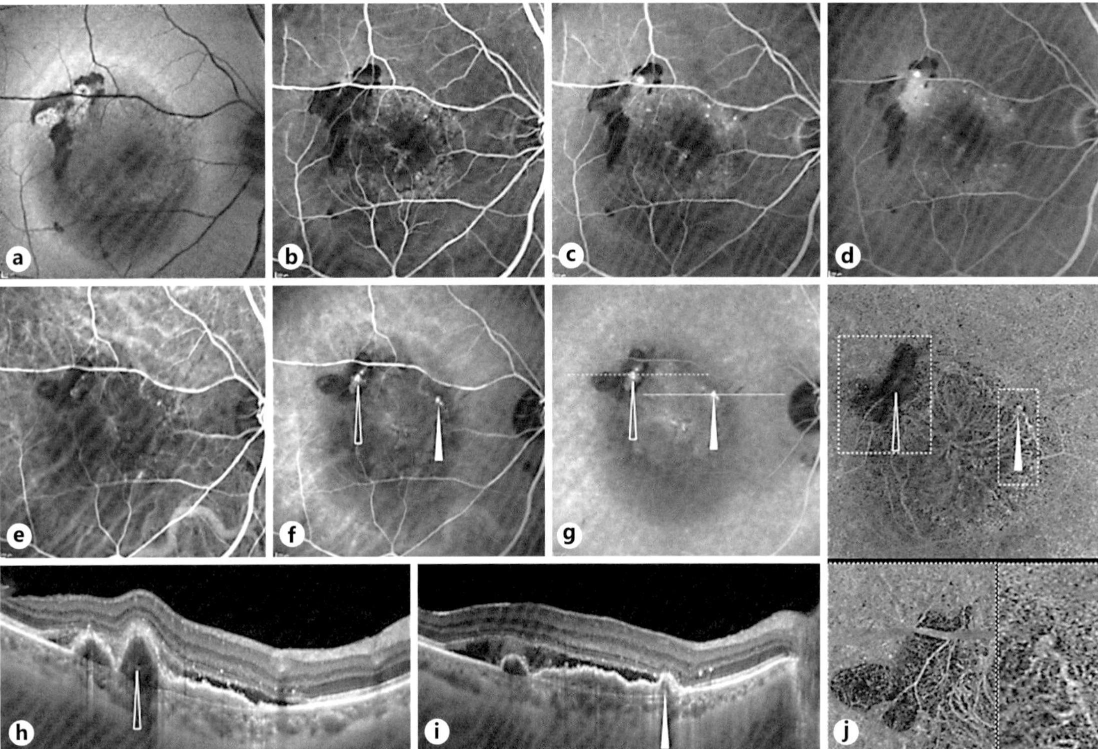

Fig. 11. Multimodal imaging of polypoidal choroidal neovascularization. **a** Fundus autofluorescence showing diffuse alteration of the retinal pigment epithelium with an area of increased signal corresponding to a subretinal hemorrhage. Fluorescein angiography in the early (**b**), middle (**c**), and late (**d**) phase displaying pinpoints of hyperfluorescence related to type 1 neovascularization. Indocyanine green angiography in the early (**e**), middle (**f**), and late (**g**) phase revealing the type 1 neovascular network with hyperfluorescent polypoidal lesions (open arrowhead and white arrowhead). White dotted line and white continuous line indicate the exact location in which the spectral domain optical coherence tomography sections were taken (**h** and **i**, respectively). Optical coherence tomography displaying detachment of retinal pigment epithelium with enlarged vessel (open arrowhead and white arrowhead) and subretinal fluid. Optical coherence tomography angiography (**j**) is able to show the central neovascular network, as type 1 neovascularization, one polypoidal lesion (white arrowhead) but not the polypoidal lesion in the temporal area (open arrowhead).

term PCV should be reserved for eyes that show paucity of the defining features of AMD, the occurrence of pachychoroid features beneath the neovascular process, and the presence of a branching vascular network with terminating polypoidal lesions (Fig. 12) [26].

Multimodal imaging techniques should be used in order to confirm the presence of polypoidal lesions. The gold standard to detect polypoidal lesions is ICGA as single or multiple focal nodular areas of hyperfluorescence arising from the choroidal circulation with or without an associated branching vascular network [27]. FA is able to show the neovascular network only in cases of large lesions and overlying atrophy of the retinal pigment epithelium. OCT reveals the polypoidal structures directly beneath the retinal pigment epithelium. The ability to detect polypoidal lesions by OCTA is not well defined. In the majority of cases, OCTA is not able to show the lesion due to

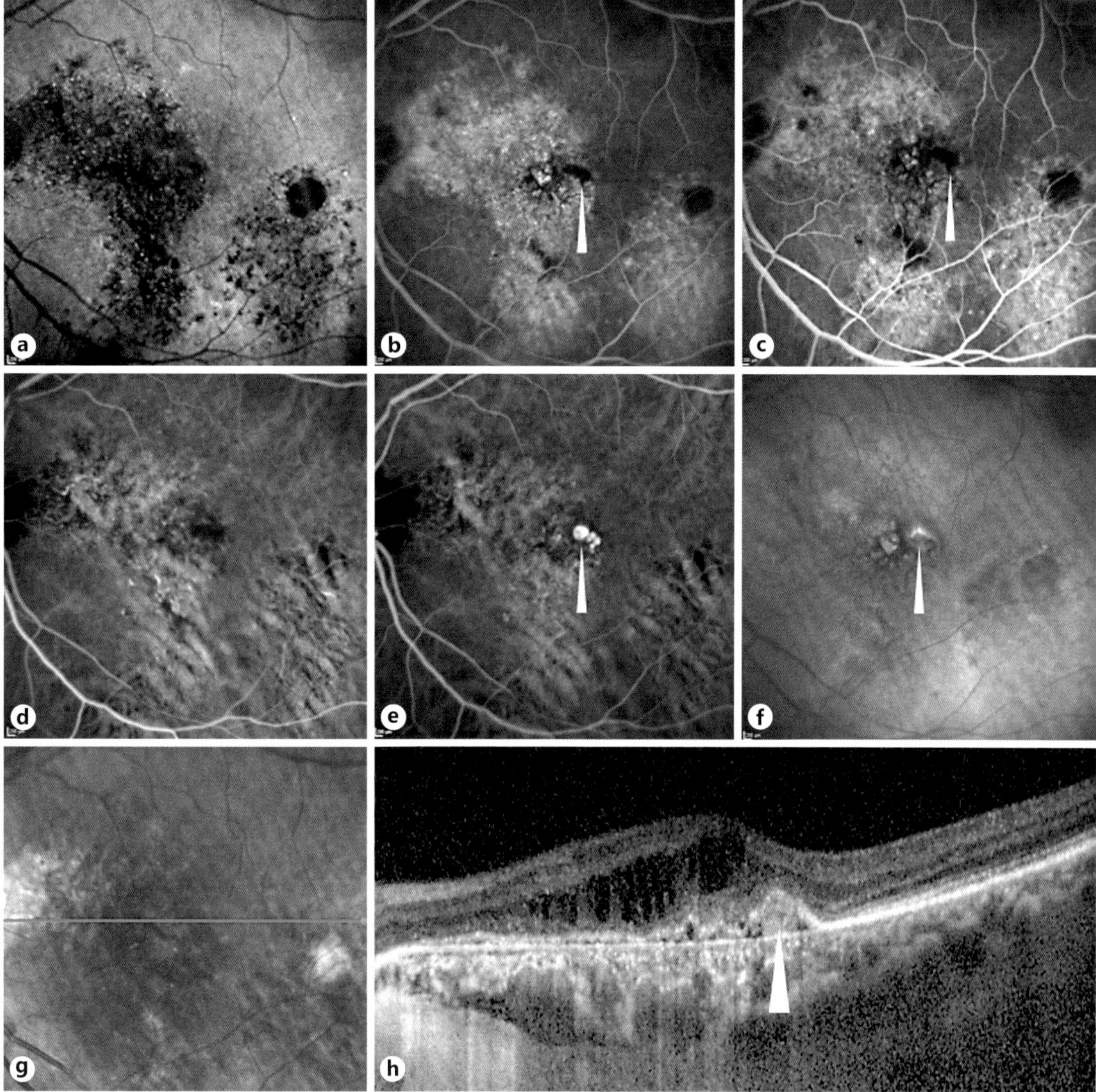

Fig. 12. Multimodal imaging of polypoidal choroidal vasculopathy. Fundus autofluorescence (**a**) showing diffuse alteration of retinal pigment epithelium and areas of atrophy. Fluorescein angiography (**b** and **c**) revealing a diffuse hyperfluorescence and hypofluorescence, and indocyanine green angiography (**d–f**) showing large choroidal vessels and focal hyperfluorescence corresponding to the polypoidal lesion (white arrowhead) with wash out in the late phase. The green line on infrared fundus photograph (**g**) indicates the exact location in which optical coherence tomography section (**h**) was taken, showing detachment of retinal pigment epithelium with enlarged vessel (white arrowhead) and intraretinal cystoid space.

the velocity of the blood flow inside and then the final appearance is an area of absence of signal.

Actually, the diagnostic criteria to confirm the presence of polypoidal lesions are: presence of early subretinal focal hyperfluorescence on ICGA (within the first 6 min), and at least one of the following criteria: nodular appearance of the polyp on stereoscopic examination, hypofluorescent halo around the nodule, presence of branching vascular network, pulsation of the polyp on dynamic ICGA, orange subretinal nodules on color fundus photography that correspond to the ICGA nodules, or massive submacular hemorrhage (≥4 disc areas in size) [28].

Geographic Atrophy

GA is a well-established end-stage manifestation of AMD. It results from the degeneration of photoreceptors, retinal pigment epithelium, and choriocapillaris [29, 30]. Color fundus photography reveals sharply delineated roughly round or oval area of hypopigmentation or depigmentation with increased visibility of the underlying choroidal vessels. On blue-light fundus autofluorescence, areas of atrophy appear as well-demarcated areas of decreased signal intensity, typically surrounded by an area of increased fundus autofluorescence signal [31]. However, in some cases, the evaluation of the foveal involvement could be challenging as the central macular luteal pigment absorbs the blue excitation light resulting in a hypoautofluorescent signal [32]. In some cases, infrared reflectance could help to identify the foveal involvement. The use of green autofluorescence eliminating the absorption by macular pigment allows the visualization of the fluorescence of the fundus under the fovea (Fig. 13).

In the early phase of FA, medium and large choroidal vessels are visible because the dye had not reached the choriocapillaris layer yet, while in the later phase, the diffusion of the fluorescein throughout the choriocapillaris leads to early obscuration of choroidal vessels and the entire area of atrophy becomes uniformly hyperfluorescent. In the early phase of ICGA, medium and large choroidal vessels are visible, and the area of atrophy progressively becomes isofluorescent and then slightly hyperfluorescent in the late phase. OCT reveals the area of hypertransmission of the signal below the level of the retinal pigment epithelium and into the choroid resulting from the loss of scatter or attenuation from the overlying retinal pigment epithelium and neurosensory retina. OCTA

shows the presence of rarefied choriocapillaris and Sattler's layer within the area atrophy [33].

It has been demonstrated that an eye with GA whose fellow eye has CNV is at significant risk for the development of CNV in the GA eye without signs of activity. Typically, CNV originated from the peripheral border of atrophy and had a final appearance of an enlarged area of GA. However, the ability to detect CNV could be challenging due to the alteration of retinal pigment epithelium and exposure of normal choroidal vessels. In this contest, OCTA is a very useful device that is able to show the neovascular network with the appropriate segmentation at the border of atrophy (Fig. 14).

In contrast to GA secondary to AMD, in patients with Stargardt disease and other retinal dystrophies, the appearance of atrophy is slightly different (Fig. 15). On fundus autofluorescence, the area of atrophy appears as hypoautofluorescent due to the absence of the retinal pigment epithelium. In the early and middle phases of FA, medium and large choroidal vessels are visible, while in the later phase borders of the area of atrophy became progressively hyperfluorescent and the center iso-hypofluorescent. ICGA reveals the area of atrophy as hypofluorescent, defined as dark atrophy, with the border more fluorescent compared with the central part [34]. OCT reveals the area of hypertransmission corresponding to the loss of the retinal pigment epithelium. OCTA shows the complete absence of choriocapillaris inside the areas of atrophy, whereas choriocapillaris lobules appear normal in density outside these regions [33].

Adult-Onset Foveomacular Vitelliform Dystrophy

The adult-onset foveomacular vitelliform dystrophy was first described by Gass in 1974 as peculiar foveomacular dystrophy and, subsequently, renamed as adult-onset foveomacular vitelliform dystrophy [35]. This term refers to an appropriate phenotype with clinical aspect, genetic compo-

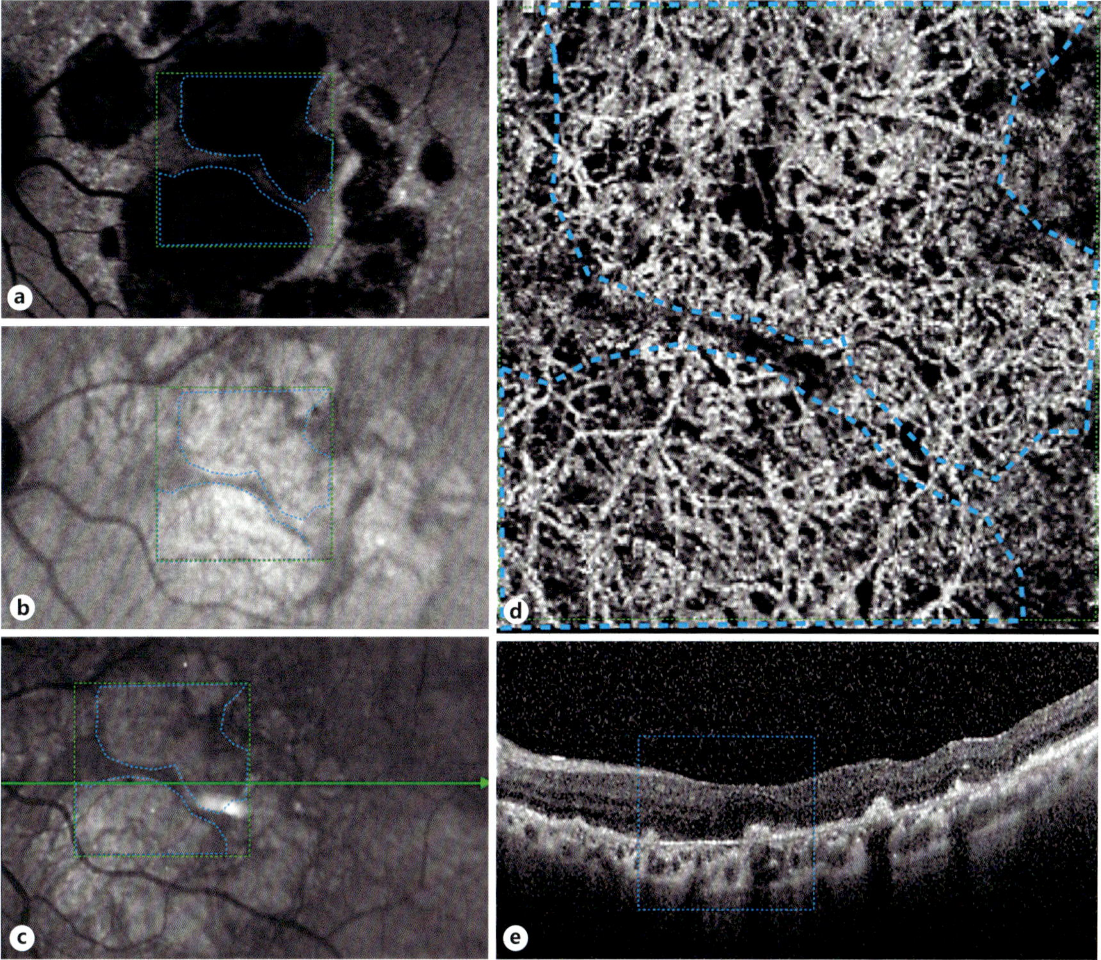

Fig. 13. Multimodal imaging of geographic atrophy. Fundus autofluorescence (**a**) and indocyanine green angiography in the late phase (**b**) showing areas of atrophy as well-demarcated areas of decreased signal intensity surrounded by areas of increased signal intensity and isofluorescence. The green line on infrared fundus photograph (**c**) indicates the exact location in which optical coherence tomography section (**e**) was taken, displaying hypertransmission of the signal below the level of the retinal pigment epithelium and into the choroid resulting from loss of scatter or attenuation from overlying retinal pigment epithelium and neurosensory retina. **d** Optical coherence tomography angiography revealing the presence of rarefied choriocapillaris and Sattler layer within the area of atrophy.

nent, and age at onset. However, the accumulation of yellowish vitelliform subretinal material has been found in various macular diseases [36]. In fact, the general term adult vitelliform lesion was introduced to describe vitelliform lesions in adults which are not necessarily of genetic origin [36]. There is controversy regarding the nature of this yellowish material as it may vary depending on the underlying clinical setting. It has been hypothesized that it probably originates from the unphagocytosed outer segment membrane [36–38]. The accumulation of this vitelliform material and, in some cases, the presence of neuroretinal detachment may be misdiagnosed as CNV.

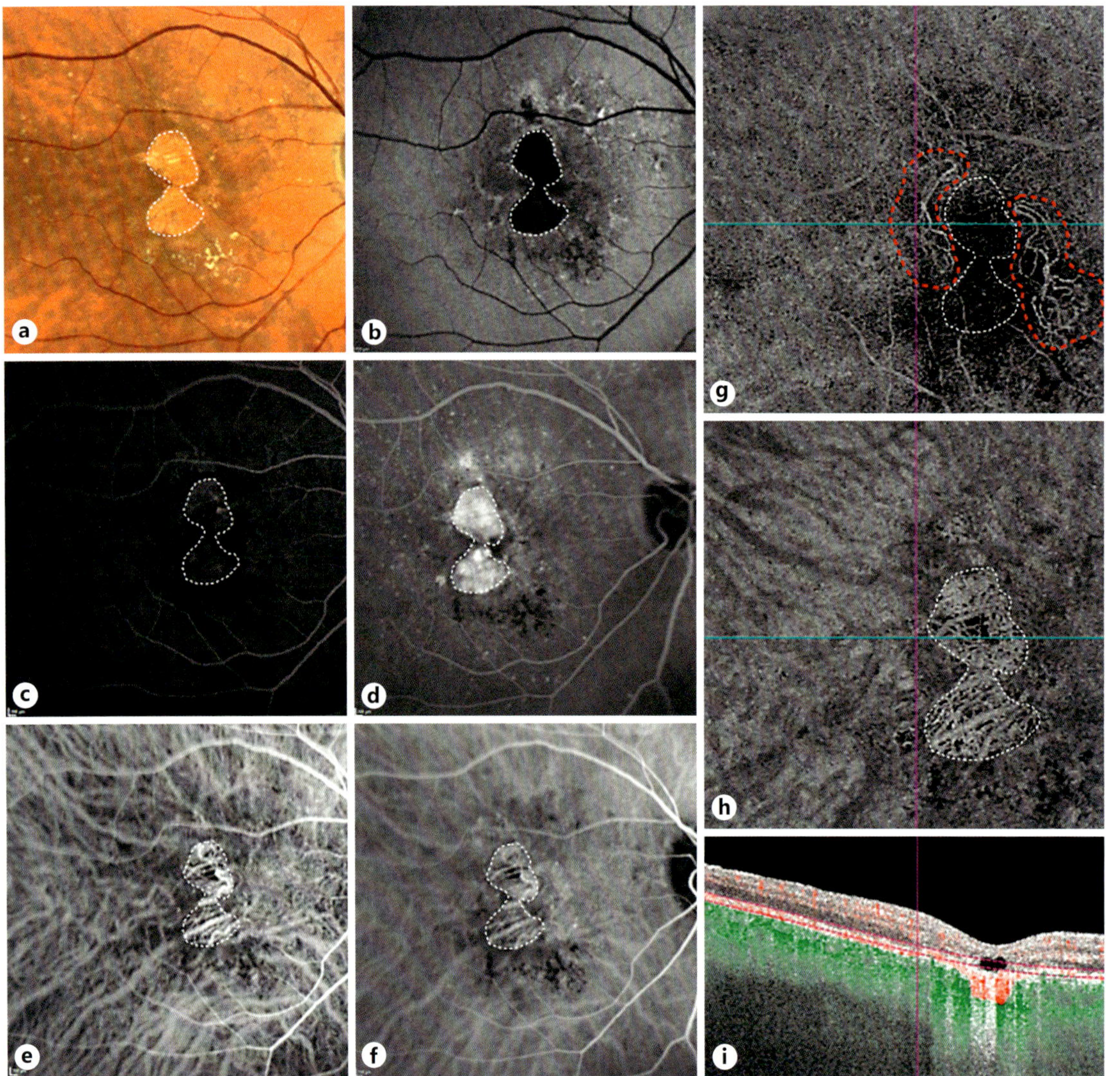

Fig. 14. Multimodal imaging of geographic atrophy complicated by choroidal neovascularization. Color fundus photography (**a**) showing the area of atrophy as an oval area of hypopigmentation or depigmentation with increased visibility of the underlying choroidal vessels, and fundus autofluorescence (**b**) as an area with decreased signal intensity (dotted white line). The early (**c**) and late phases (**d**) of fluorescein angiography revealing a central hyperfluorescence with staining. **e**, **f** Indocyanine green angiography displaying well evidently the medium-large choroidal vessels under the atrophic area. Optical coherence tomography angiography at choriocapillaris segmentation (**g**) showing 2 neovascular networks at the peripheral border of atrophy, and at the choroid segmentation (**h**) a rarefied choriocapillaris and Sattler layer within the area atrophy with enhanced view of choroidal vessels. **i** Optical coherence tomography displaying the hypertransmission of the signal below the atrophic area.

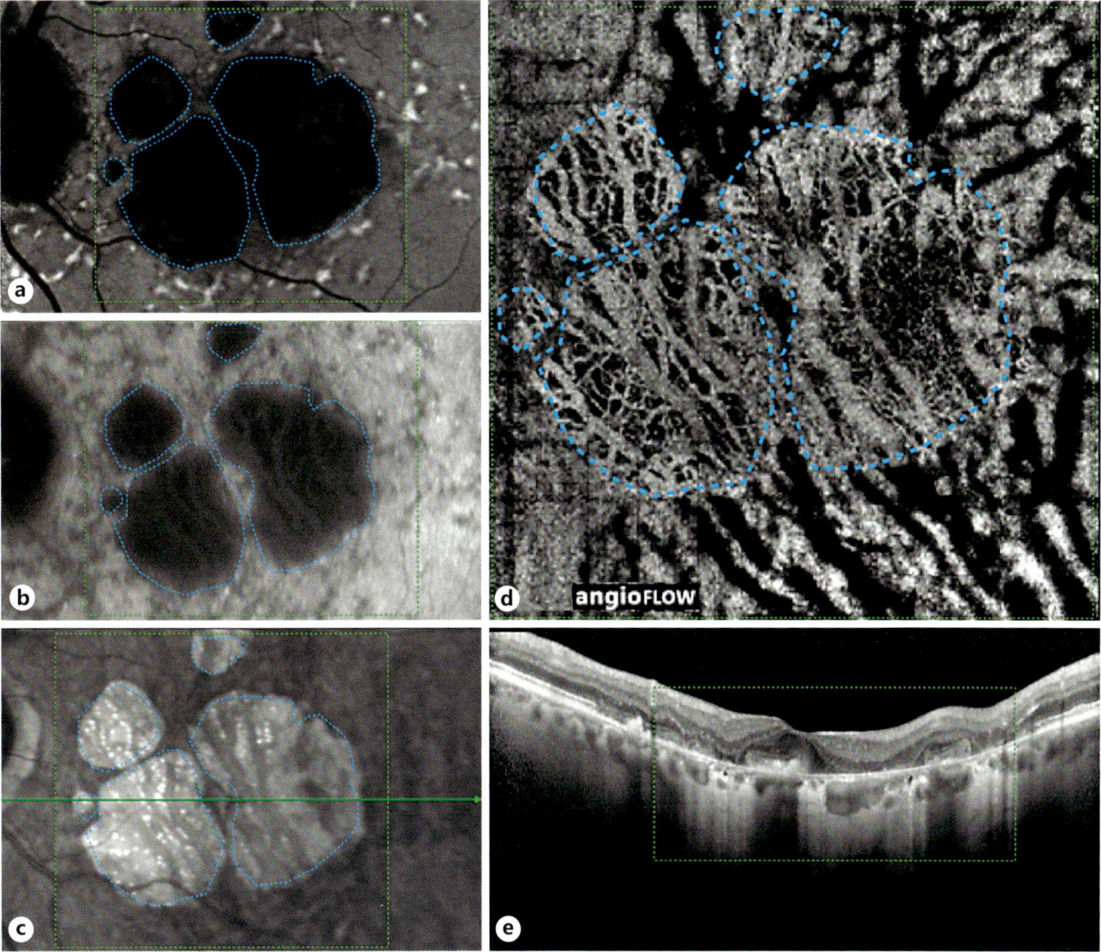

Fig. 15. Multimodal imaging of atrophy secondary to Stargardt disease. **a** Fundus autofluorescence showing areas of atrophy as well-demarcated areas of decreased signal intensity. **b** The late phase of indocyanine green angiography revealing central hypofluorescent areas, defined as dark atrophy. The green line on infrared fundus photograph (**c**) indicates the exact location where optical coherence tomography section (**e**) was taken, displaying hypertransmission of the signal below the level of the retinal pigment epithelium and into the choroid resulting from loss of scatter or attenuation from overlying retinal pigment epithelium and neurosensory retina. **d** Optical coherence tomography angiography revealing the complete absence of choriocapillaris inside the areas of atrophy, whereas choriocapillaris lobules appear normal in density outside these regions.

Fundus color photography, typically, shows the presence of a whitish-yellow vitelliform lesion corresponding to the hyperautofluorescent appearance on fundus autofluorescence (Fig. 16). This material appears hyperreflective on infrared reflectance, hypofluorescent on FA in the early phase and then hyperfluorescent from the edges towards the center in the late phase; on ICGA, it appears hypofluorescent in both the early and late phases due to the masking effect. OCT displays the lesion as hyperreflective between the retinal pigment epithelium and the ellipsoid zone of the photoreceptors. Sometimes, these lesions may be complicated by CNV, and the diagnosis could be

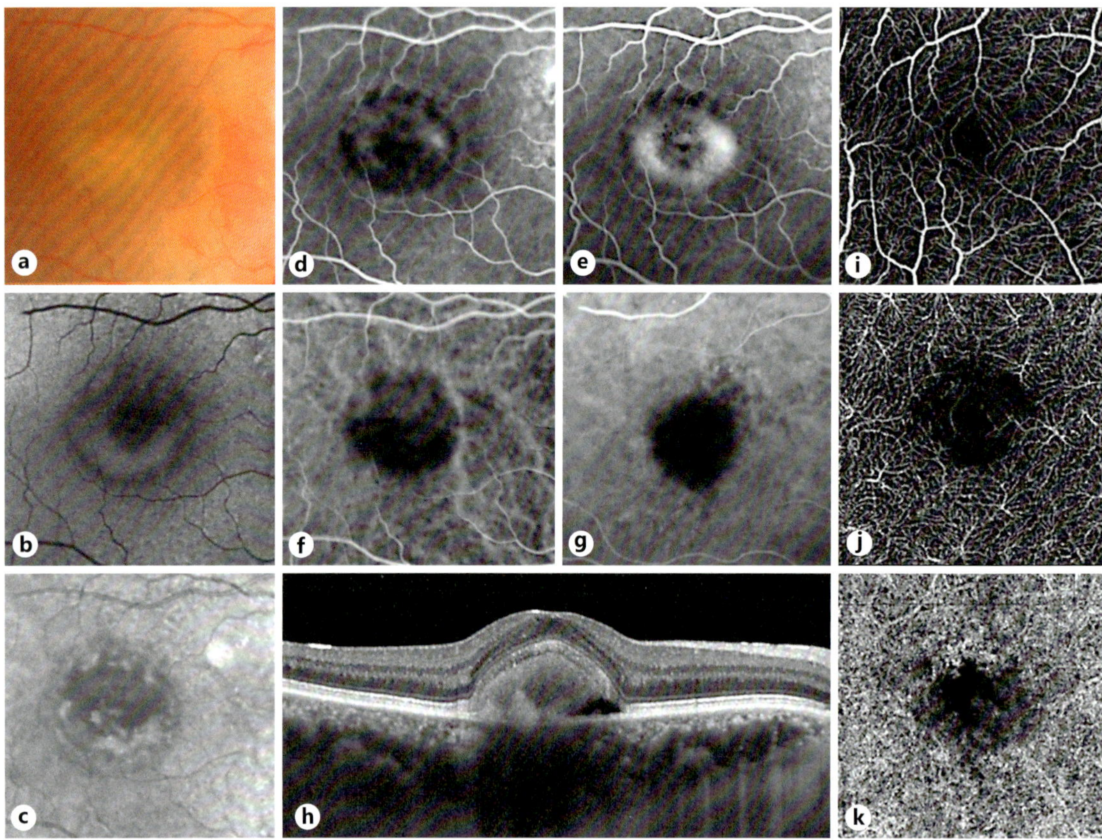

Fig. 16. Multimodal imaging of adult-onset foveomacular vitelliform dystrophy. Color fundus photography (**a**), fundus autofluorescence (**b**), and infrared reflectance (**c**) showing the central yellowish, hyperautofluorescent, and hyper-hyporeflective vitelliform lesion. Fluorescein angiography revealing a hypofluorescent area in the early phase (**d**) that becomes hyperfluorescent from the edges towards the center in the later phases (**e**). Indocyanine green angiography displaying a central hypofluorescent area in both early (**f**) and late phases (**g**). **h** Spectral domain optical coherence tomography showing the the hyperreflective material between retinal pigment epithelium and the ellipsoid zone of the photoreceptors. Optical coherence tomography angiography revealing the displacement of blood vessels at both the superficial (**i**) and more evidently at deep capillary plexuses (**j**). **k** Choriocapillaris segmentation showing a round dark area corresponding to the limits of the vitelliform material due to limitation of light penetration.

challenging. A combination of clinical assessment and multimodal imaging is necessary to confirm or exclude the CNV.

Idiopathic Macular Telangiectasia

Idiopathic perifoveal or juxtafoveolar retinal telangiectasia is retinal capillary ectasia limited to the perifoveal area without any apparent specific cause [39]. According to the Gass classification, idiopathic macular telangiectasias are divided into 4 groups: group 1 – a less severe form of Coats disease characterized by unilateral parafoveal retinal telangiectasia; group 2 – bilateral symmetric juxtafoveolar telangiectasia affecting the temporal half of the juxtafoveolar areas with minimal intraretinal exudation; group 3 – bilateral parafoveolar telangiectasia with minimal intraretinal exudation; group 4 – familial optic disc

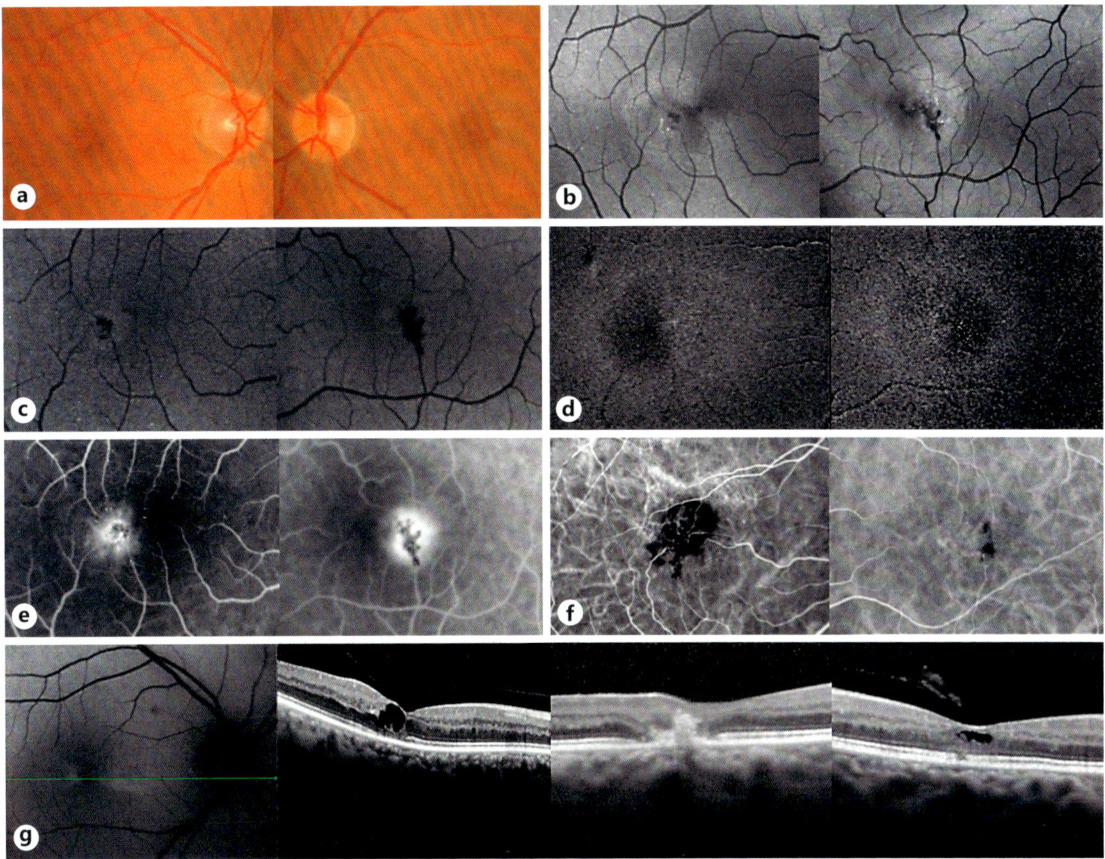

Fig. 17. Multimodal imaging of idiopathic macular telangiectasia. **a** Color fundus photography revealing the abnormal mild discoloration near the fovea with multiple golden crystalline refractile deposits. Confocal blue reflectance (**b**), blue autofluorescence (**c**) and macular pigment measurment with fundus autofluorescence (**d**) showing the abnormal pigment disposition. **e** Fluorescein angiography displaying the dilated telangiectatic perifoveal vessels with right angles course and mild leakage. **f** Indocyanine green angiography showing an hypofluorescent area due to masking of macular pigment. **g** Optical coherence tomography on fundus autofluorescence revealing the intra-retinal hyporeflective spaces in the retina with remodeling of outer and inner retinal layers.

pallor and perifoveolar retinal capillary occlusion [39].

Later, this classification was modified dividing these lesions into 3 groups and each group was subdivided into 2 subgroups. In particular, group 1A was defined as visible and exudative lesions; group 1B as visible, exudative, and focal telangiectasia; group 2A as occult and nonexudative telangiectasia; group 2B as juvenile occult familial telangiectasia; group 3A as occlusive with minimal exudation; group 3B as occlusive lesions associated with central nervous system vasculopathy [40]. Subsequently, Yannuzzi et al. [41] proposed a new classification in which type 1 telangiectasia was defined as aneurysmal telangiectasia and type 2 (Mac Tel 2) as perifoveal idiopathic macular telangiectasia.

Typically, Mac Tel 2 is bilateral, temporal, and symmetrical; however, there have been reports of unilateral, asymmetric, and asymptomatic cases [42]. It has been hypothesized that the primary involvement is the alteration of Müller cells and the secondary involvement is vascular and tissue remodeling [39–41]. The earliest ophthalmoscopic changes are a mild grayish discoloration of the retina with loss of retinal transparency temporal to the fovea and later the presence of multiple golden crystalline refractile deposits near the inner retinal surface (Fig. 17). Confocal blue fundus reflectance autofluorescence reveals an increased signal at the foveal region due to macular pigment depletion, starting from the temporal side [43]. FA shows the capillary telangiectasia with dilated and blunted retinal venules at right angles into the temporal parafoveolar area. OCT reveals the outer retinal atrophy as thinning and loss of the normal outer retinal architecture with intraretinal hyporeflective spaces and highly reflective intraretinal areas as large vessel dilation. The focal atrophy of the foveolar retina may create a lamellar macular hole and full thickness macular hole due to the Müller cell degeneration [41, 44]. Idiopathic macular telangiectasia could be complicated by retinal choroidal anastomosis, visible on ICGA and OCTA [45].

References

1 Novais EA, Baumal CR, Sarraf D, Freund KB, Duker JS: Multimodal imaging in retinal disease: a consensus definition. Ophthalmic Surg Lasers Imaging Retina 2016;47:201–205.

2 Madonna R, Cevik C, Cocco N: Multimodality imaging for pre-clinical assessment of Fabry's cardiomyopathy. Eur Heart J Cardiovasc Imaging 2014;15:1094–1100.

3 Creuzot-Garcher C, Martin-Phipps T, Beynat J, Astruc K, Brassac K, Bron AM: Effectiveness of a mobile diabetic retinopathy screening campaign to encourage diabetics to undergo regular ophthalmic follow-up. Ophthalmic Res 2014;52:206–211.

4 Tan AC, Fleckenstein M, Schmitz-Valckenberg S, Holz FG: Clinical application of multicolor imaging technology. Ophthalmologica 2016;236:8–18.

5 Delori FC, Goger DG, Dorey CK: Age-related accumulation and spatial distribution of lipofuscin in RPE of normal subjects. Invest Ophthalmol Vis Sci 2001;42:1855–1866.

6 Holz FG, Bellman C, Staudt S, Schütt F, Völcker HE: Fundus autofluorescence and development of geographic atrophy in age-related macular degeneration. Invest Ophthalmol Vis Sci 2001;42:1051–1056.

7 Holz FG, Bindewald-Wittich A, Fleckenstein M, Dreyhaupt J, Scholl HP, Schmitz-Valckenberg S; FAM-Study Group: Progression of geographic atrophy and impact of fundus autofluorescence patterns in age-related macular degeneration. Am J Ophthalmol 2007;143:463–472.

8 Chakravarthy U, Walsh AC, Muldrew A, Updike PG, Barbour T, Sadda SR: Quantitative fluorescein angiographic analysis of choroidal neovascular membranes: validation and correlation with visual function. Invest Ophthalmol Vis Sci 2007;48:349–354.

9 Yannuzzi LA, Sorenson JA, Guyer DR, Slakter JS, Chang B, Orlock D: Indocyanine green videoangiography: current status. Eur J Ophthalmol 1994;4:69–81.

10 Huang D, Swanson EA, Lin CP, Schuman JS, Stinson WG, Chang W, Hee MR, Flotte T, Gregory K, Puliafito CA, et al: Optical coherence tomography. Science 1991;254:1178–1181.

11 Spaide RF, Klancnik JM Jr, Cooney MJ: Retinal vascular layers imaged by fluorescein angiography and optical coherence tomography angiography. JAMA Ophthalmol 2015;133:45–50.

12 Matsunaga D, Yi J, Puliafito CA, Kashani AH: OCT angiography in healthy human subjects. Ophthalmic Surg Lasers Imaging Retina 2014;45:510–515.

13 Gass JD: Stereoscopic Atlas of Macular Diseases, ed 4. St Louis, CV Mosby, 1997, pp 26–30.

14 Fernandes LH, Freund KB, Yannuzzi LA, et al: The nature of focal areas of hyperfluorescence or hot spots imaged with indocyanine green angiography. Retina 2002;22:557–568.

15 Staurenghi G, Orzalesi N, La Capria A, Aschero M: Laser treatment of feeder vessels in subfoveal choroidal neovascular membranes: a revisitation using dynamic indocyanine green angiography. Ophthalmology 1998;105:2297–2305.

16 Spaide RF, Fujimoto JG, Waheed NK, Sadda SR, Staurenghi G: Optical coherence tomography angiography. Prog Retin Eye Res DOI: 10.1016/j.preteyeres.2017.11.003.

17 Gass JD: Biomicroscopic and histopathologic considerations regarding the feasibility of surgical excision of subfoveal neovascular membranes. Am J Ophthalmol 1994;118:258–298.

18 Giani A, Luiselli C, Esmaili DD, Salvetti P, Cigada M, Miller JW, Staurenghi G: Spectral-domain optical coherence tomography as an indicator of fluorescein angiography leakage from choroidal neovascularization. Invest Ophthalmol Vis Sci 2011;52:5579–5586.

19 Hartnett ME, Weiter JJ, Staurenghi G, Elsner AE: Deep retinal vascular anomalous complexes in advanced age-related macular degeneration. Ophthalmology 1996;103:2042–2053.

20 Yannuzzi LA, Negrão S, Iida T, Carvalho C, Rodriguez-Coleman H, Slakter J, Freund KB, Sorenson J, Orlock D, Borodoker N: Retinal angiomatous proliferation in age-related macular degeneration. Retina 2001;21:416–434.

21 Gass JD, Agarwal A, Lavina AM, Tawansy KA: Focal inner retinal hemorrhages in patients with drusen: an early sign of occult choroidal neovascularization and chorioretinal anastomosis. Retina 2003; 23:741–751.

22 Freund KB, Ho IV, Barbazetto IA, Koizumi H, Laud K, Ferrara D, Matsumoto Y, Sorenson JA, Yannuzzi L: Type 3 neovascularization: the expanded spectrum of retinal angiomatous proliferation. Retina 2008;28:201–211.

23 Freund KB, Zweifel SA, Engelbert M: Do we need a new classification for choroidal neovascularization in age-related macular degeneration? Retina 2010;30: 1333–1349.

24 Yannuzzi LA, Freund KB, Takahashi BS: Review of retinal angiomatous proliferation or type 3 neovascularization. Retina 2008;28:375–384.

25 Yannuzzi LA, Sorenson J, Spaide RF, Lipson B: Idiopathic polypoidal choroidal vasculopathy (IPCV). Retina 1990; 10:1–8.

26 Balaratnasingam C, Lee WK, Koizumi H, Dansingani K, Inoue M, Freund KB: Polypoidal choroidal vasculopathy: a distinct disease or manifestation of many? Retina 2016;36:1.

27 Shiraga F, Matsuo T, Yokoe S, et al: Surgical treatment of submacular hemorrhage associated with idiopathic polypoidal choroidal vasculopathy. Am J Ophthalmol 1999;128:147–154.

28 Koh A, Lee WK, Chen LJ, et al: EVEREST study: efficacy and safety of verteporfin photodynamic therapy in combination with ranibizumab or alone versus ranibizumab monotherapy in patients with symptomatic macular polypoidal choroidal vasculopathy. Retina 2012;32: 1453–1464.

29 Ferris 3rd FL, Wilkinson CP, Bird A, et al: Clinical classification of age-related macular degeneration. Ophthalmology 2013;120:844–851.

30 Holz FG, Strauss EC, Schmitz-Valckenberg S, van Lookeren Campagne M: Geographic atrophy: clinical features and potential therapeutic approaches. Ophthalmology 2014;121:1079–1091.

31 von Ruckmann A, Fitzke FW, Bird AC: Distribution of fundus autofluorescence with a scanning laser ophthalmoscope. Br J Ophthalmol 1995;79:407–412.

32 Lindner M, Boker A, Mauschitz MM, et al: Directional kinetics of geographic atrophy progression in age-related macular degeneration with foveal sparing. Ophthalmology 2015;122:1356–1365.

33 Pellegrini M, Acquistapace A, Oldani M, Cereda MG, Giani A, Cozzi M, Staurenghi G: Dark atrophy: an optical coherence tomography angiography study. Ophthalmology 2016;123:1879–1886.

34 Giani A, Pellegrini M, Carini E, Peroglio Deiro A, Bottoni F, Staurenghi G: The dark atrophy with indocyanine green angiography in Stargardt disease. Invest Ophthalmol Vis Sci 2012;53:3999–4004.

35 Gass J: A clinicopathologic study of a peculiar foveomacular dystrophy. Trans Am Ophthalmol Soc 1974;72:139–156.

36 Freund KB, Laud K, Lima LH, Spaide RF, Zweifel S, Yannuzzi LA: Acquired vitelliform lesions: correlation of clinical findings and multiple imaging analyses. Retina 2011;31:13–25.

37 Dubovy SR, Hairston RJ, Schatz H, Schachat AP, Bressler NM, Finkelstein D, Green WR: Adult-onset foveomacular pigment epithelial dystrophy: clinicopathologic correlation of three cases. Retina 2000;20:638–649.

38 Arnold JJ, Sarks JP, Killingsworth MC, Kettle EK, Sarks SH: Adult vitelliform macular degeneration: a clinicopathological study. Eye (Lond) 2003;17:717–726.

39 Gass JD, Oyakawa RT: Idiopathic juxtafoveolar retinal telangiectasis. Arch Ophthalmol 1982;100:769–780.

40 Gass JD, Blodi BA: Idiopathic juxtafoveolar retinal telangiectasis. Update of classification and follow-up study. Ophthalmology 1993;100:1536–1546.

41 Yannuzzi LA, Bardal AM, Freund KB, et al: Idiopathic macular telangiectasia. Arch Ophthalmol 2006;124:450–460.

42 Wong WT, Forooghian F, Majumdar Z, et al: Fundus autofluorescence in type 2 idiopathic macular telangiectasia: correlation with optical coherence tomography and microperimetry. Am J Ophthalmol 2009;148:573–583.

43 Charbel Issa P, Berendschot TT, Staurenghi G, Holz FG, Scholl HP: Confocal blue reflectance imaging in type 2 idiopathic macular telangiectasia. Invest Ophthalmol Vis Sci 2008;49:1172–1177.

44 Charbel Issa P, Scholl HP, Gaudric A, et al: Macular full-thickness and lamellar holes in association with type 2 idiopathic macular telangiectasia. Eye (Lond) 2009;23:435–441.

45 Balaratnasingam C, Yannuzzi LA, Spaide RF: Possible choroidal neovascularization in macular telangiectasia type 2. Retina 2015;35:2317–2322.

Federico Corvi
ASST Fatebenefratelli Sacco
Via G.B. Grassi, 74
20157 Milan (Italy)
E-Mail federico.corvi@yahoo.it

Subject Index